MENTAL ILLNESS AND SOCIAL POLICY

THE AMERICAN EXPERIENCE

MENTAL ILLNESS AND SOCIAL POLICY

THE AMERICAN EXPERIENCE

AN INQUIRY

CONCERNING

THE DISEASES AND FUNCTIONS

OF

THE BRAIN,

THE SPINAL CORD,

AND

THE NERVES

BY

AMARIAH BRIGHAM

ARNO PRESS
A NEW YORK TIMES COMPANY
New York • 1973

Reprint Edition 1973 by Arno Press Inc.

MENTAL ILLNESS AND SOCIAL POLICY:
  The American Experience
ISBN for complete set: 0-405-05190-5
See last pages of this volume for titles.

Manufactured in the United States of America

———————◆———————

Library of Congress Cataloging in Publication Data

Brigham, Amariah, 1798-1849.
    An inquiry concerning the diseases and functions of
the brain, the spinal cord, and the nerves.

    (Mental illness and social policy: the American
experience)
    Reprint of the ed. published by G. Adlard, New York.
    1. Brain--Diseases.   2. Spinal cord--Diseases.
3. Nervous systems--Diseases.   I. Title.
II. Series.   [DNLM: WL B855i 1840F]
RC341.B8 1973   616.8   73-2388
ISBN 0-405-05196-4

AN INQUIRY

CONCERNING

THE DISEASES AND FUNCTIONS

OF

THE BRAIN,

THE SPINAL CORD,

AND

THE NERVES.

BY

AMARIAH BRIGHAM, M. D.

NEW-YORK.
GEORGE ADLARD, 168 BROADWAY.
1840.

Printed by
ELIHU GEER,
HARTFORD, CONN.

PREFACE.

THE object of the following work is to call the attention of those practitioners of medicine into whose hands it falls, to the importance of the nervous system ; and to persuade them to embrace every opportunity that is presented, for studying its functions and diseases.

For this purpose I have endeavored to give a partial summary of what is now known respecting this system. I have collected a large number of cases explanatory of its diseases and functions — cases that are scattered through many volumes, to which I have added a consider, able number that have fallen under my own observation ; and have thus sought to indicate the way that this system should be studied in order to increase our knowl. edge of its functions and our means of remedying its diseases.

In the second part I have briefly treated of a number of diseases the pathology of which is not yet settled. I have not sought to give full accounts of these, but to direct attention to a few important circumstances and such as require further investigation.

Affections of the nervous system have always existed,

and always formed a considerable proportion of the diseases, and those the most obscure, by which the human
system has been assailed.

But they have vastly increased with the increase of
civilization, and now constitute a far greater proportion of the diseases of mankind, than in past ages, and
consequently demand far more attention.   If this volume
induces but a few, to investigate the affections of this
system with care, to record and make known the facts
they observe and thus add something to our knowledge
of its functions and diseases, it will be all that the author
expects.

Hartford, Ct., Jan. 1st, 1840.

CONTENTS.

Part I.

Part II.

DISEASES OF THE BRAIN, AND OF OTHER PARTS OF THE NERVOUS SYSTEM.

Appendix.

Note A.

Note B.

DISEASES

OF

THE BRAIN,

ET C. ET C.

Part I.

GENERAL OBSERVATIONS ON THE STUDY OF THE STRUC- TURE AND FUNCTIONS OF THE BRAIN.

THE obvious though mysterious connection between the brain and the mind — between the large mass of matter within the skull and our spiritual nature, has given rise to much investigation and controversy.

But many of the investigations and controversies relating to this subject, have not, I apprehend, been conducted in a right spirit, with the sole desire of ascertaining the exact truth, but oftener with a wish to establish, or to overthrow, some preconceived and frequently pre-advanced opinion.

I hope the reader of these observations will endeavor to divest himself of all prejudices upon the subject, and examine, one by one, and with rigid impartiality the various methods which have been recommended by writers, to determine what are the functions of the brain. Such an examination seems to be necessary at the outset, that we may ascertain satisfactorily to ourselves,

2

which of the methods proposed will be most profitable for us to pursue.

We should also call to mind that but little is now known upon this subject; that all physiologists of reputation and candor admit, that though no other subject is more deserving of thorough investigation, yet there has been but a small amount of evidence furnished, to enable us to determine with accuracy the office, or use. of the various parts of the brain of man. It therefore devolves upon the anatomists, physiologists and pathologists of the present generation, to make investigations upon this important subject to a far greater extent than have hitherto been made, in order to dispel the darkness, in which it is at present involved.

And it is gratifying to perceive that the functions of the brain and nerves are now attracting the attention of medical inquirers, much more than at any former period. Many of the most industrious and distinguished members of the medical profession, and such as from official station and other advantages have the best opportunities for investigating such subjects, are prosecuting inquiries with great earnestness respecting the growth, structure, and diseased appearance of the brain and nerves, with a view of ascertaining their functions and remedying their diseases. We may therefore reasonably expect within a short period valuable additions to our knowledge of the nervous system. We are encouraged in this belief from the important facts which have been made known within a few years by the labors of Gall, Reil, Spurzheim, Flourens, Bell, Magendie, Foville, Lallemand, Abercrombie, Andral, Serres, Tenneman, Muller, Hall, Solly, Grainger, &c., who, with many others, have cultivated this department of medical inquiry. These distinguished men have not pursued the same methods of investigation; some have had recourse to experiments upon the living

nervous system ; others have chiefly devoted their attention to its diseased condition and to noticing the symptoms
produced by this condition ; while others have watched
its growth and development, and marked the manifestation of function at different periods ; and from these dissimilar methods of investigation, we have within a few
years been put in possession of more knowledge respecting the nervous system, than had come down to us from
all previous time.

The study of the human brain yields in utility and
dignity to none other. It is the study of the most important part of our organization, of that portion for which
all the others seem to be created. It is also of the highest
philosophical interest, from the connection of the nervous
system with the manifestation of mental phenomena. I
am fully convinced that this system plays a more important part in the human organization than is generally supposed, and that its influence in causing, continuing and
even curing disease has been too much disregarded. It
is by this system that all impressions are perceived, and
all knowledge of surrounding objects derived, and by
which we can know either pleasure or pain. It is universally distributed to the body — to every organ, to
every muscle and to every fibre, endowing these parts
with sensation, life and energy, and with the power of
acting in harmony.

From the general diffusion of this system and its known
uses, we should expect it to have great influence in disease, and that as intelligence and mental cultivation, the
excitement of the feelings and passions, all of which affect
this system, increase, that an increase of nervous diseases and new affections of this system should be observed. And this we find to be true. Apoplexy, palsy,
inflammation of the brain, dropsy of the head, insanity,
&c., are far more common now than in past ages, and

are most observed in countries where there is the most mental excitement. We also now witness forms of nervous disease, or affections of the brain and nerves that were nearly unknown half a century since, such as tic doloreux and delirium tremens, which have recently become as common diseases as any we are called upon to remedy. It is therefore incumbent upon the practical physicians and surgeons of the present day, to give increased attention to the study of the nervous system — to ascertain and make known the functions of its various parts, in order to qualify themselves to the best of their ability to remedy or to prevent its diseases.

In the first place, an accurate knowledge of the anatomy of the brain is necessary. Its structure should be carefully examined, and its connection with the nerves, with the skull, the membranes and blood-vessels, be noticed and remembered. Possessed of this knowledge physicians will be less likely to err in prognosis and in the treatment of the diseases of this organ, and above all, they will be able, whenever such diseases prove fatal, to ascertain and to describe to others their exact location, extent, and connection. This knowledge, together with the history of the symptoms, will aid essentially in determining the functions of the parts affected. In this manner every practitioner may do something to lessen the obscurity that now exists respecting the functions of the brain and nerves, and aid in increasing our knowledge of their diseases.

But I regret to say, that generally diseases of the nervous system are not thus investigated. If the brain is examined after death, it is often done in so hurried and coarse a manner, and so little is known of its healthy appearance, and structure, and connections, that important facts are overlooked. If considerable effusion into the lateral ventricles is observed, this is frequently deemed the cause of death and no further or minute examination is made. Attempts to elucidate the diseases of the spinal marrow by autopsical examination are quite rare, and of those of the ganglionic system still more so. I am aware that such neglect of the nervous system is not absolutely general, but I am convinced it is nearly so throughout most of the country.*

I am the more anxious to remedy this neglect of examining the condition of the brain and nerves, because I look to this method — to facts derived from the examination of the diseased appearance of the nervous system, in connection with the history of the symptoms — as one of the most important methods for obtaining a knowledge of the functions of the various parts of this system.

---

* We have occasional accounts of autopsical examinations made in the hospitals of large cities, and of some few in private practice; but how small the number of these observations compared with those that would be furnished if such examinations were common throughout the country. There are probably about 20,000 physicians in the United States. If their attention could be earnestly and properly directed to the subject we are considering, how rapidly would our knowledge of the functions of the nervous system and of its diseases be increased. Considering the importance of minutely studying the nervous system, every physician should embrace all the opportunities presented him for this purpose. He should supply himself with a few instruments expressly for autopsical examinations — a few knives, a small saw, hammer and large screw-driver or iron lever, a small gimblet and pincers, some copper wire, scales and weights, needles, thread, sponges and comb. These will enable him to make the requisite examination and to restore the parts without disfiguring the body. Attention to this last particular is very important, as it serves to remove most of the objections made by friends to such investigations. It is possible to remove the brain without disfiguring the forehead. This may be accomplished by sawing across the frontal bone, three inches above the eye brows from one temple to the other, and meeting a circular cut through the lateral and posterior parts of the skull.

2*

Every one knows that certain symptoms indicate disease of the brain, or its membranes, or nerves ; but until quite recently, and now almost generally, physicians rest satisfied with merely knowing that the disease is located somewhere within the skull. But we should certainly strive to know more than this, and I feel confident that by numerous and careful observations we may be able to determine from the symptoms, not merely that the disease is within the skull, but whether the membranes, or nerves, or the substance of the brain is affected, and often what part of this latter organ and what nerves are diseased. Few physicians are now satisfied with merely knowing that a patient has some disease within the abdomen or thorax ; they seek to know what particular organ is affected, and what tissue or portion of the organ is diseased, and this knowledge they can generally obtain by a thorough examination of the case, and comparing the symptoms manifested with those exhibited by others where examination after death revealed the connection between the symptoms and the organic disease. But much of this knowledge — of this ability to determine the exact location of the disease within the abdomen, or chest — is of modern origin ; and we have but to pursue the same course as regards diseases of the nervous system, in order to judge from the symptoms what portion of it is affected. This field of investigation is indeed very great, and will require for a long time many laborers, but ultimately, I apprehend, will richly reward those who cultivate it.

SECTION I.

STRUCTURE OF THE BRAIN, &C.

BY the brain I mean all the mass contained within the cranium and which it entirely fills. The weight of this mass in adult white males, varies from 3 lbs. 2 oz. to 4 lbs. 6 oz. troy — the weight I uniformly mean, except when avoirdupois is expressly mentioned.

The brain of men greatly distinguished for their intellectual power is usually large. That of Cuvier was one third larger than an ordinary adult brain. It weighed 4 lbs. 11 oz. 4 drachms and 30 grains ; that of Dupuytren 4 lbs. 10 oz. According to Desmoulins the brain decreases in weight after the age of seventy. The female brain is lighter than that of the male, usually from four to eight ounces. It varies from 2 lbs. 8 oz. to 3 lbs. 10 oz. "I never found," says Tiedeman, from whom the above statements are derived, "a female brain that weighed four pounds."*

The following elaborate table by Dr. Simns,† contains the results of examinations instituted to ascertain the average weight of the healthy brain at different periods of life. The estimates it will be noticed are by avoirdupois.

---

* On the brain of the negro compared with that of the European and the ourang-outang. By Professor Tiedeman, of Heidelberg. Philosophical Transactions for 1836. Part II.

† Medico-chirurgical Transactions. Vol. 19.

Years.	Number weighed.	Average.
1 to 2	9	2 lb. 1 oz. nearly.
2 " 3	3	2 " $4\frac{1}{3}$ "
3 " 4	5	2 " $6\frac{1}{5}$ "
4 " 5	3	2 " 7 "
5 " 10	9	2 " $8\frac{4}{9}$ "
10 " 15	14	2 " $12\frac{4}{14}$ "
15 " 20	3	2 " 13 "
20 " 30	19	2 " $12\frac{14}{19}$ "
30 " 40	22	2 " $13\frac{14}{22}$ "
40 " 50	29	2 " $14\frac{20}{29}$ "
50 " 60	35	2 " $13\frac{2}{35}$ "
60 " 70	42	2 " $11\frac{34}{42}$ "
70 and upwards	44	2 " $10\frac{5}{44}$ "

" The inference from this table is, that the average weight of the brain goes on increasing from one year old to twenty, between twenty and thirty there is a slight decrease in the average, afterwards it increases and arrives at a maximum between forty and fifty ; after fifty to old age the brain gradually decreases in weight."

This account respecting the increase and decrease in the weight of the brain is, I presume, in the main correct, though sometimes the head continues to increase in size, long after the period mentioned. Of this I have been assured by those who have measured at different periods after adult age, the heads of men distinguished for intellectual power and energy. Dr. Spurzheim informed me that he measured the heads of several distinguished men, during his visit to England in 1814, and twelve years after re-measured them, and found they had increased considerably. Some of these individuals were above forty years of age at the time of the first measurement, but had devoted themselves with ardor to intellectual pursuits during the interval.

" This phenomenon," says M. Itard,* " is not rare in the adult, especially among men given to study, or profound meditation, or who devote themselves, without relaxation, to the agitations of an unquiet and enterprising spirit. Bonaparte may be cited as an example. His head was not large in early life, but acquired in after years a development nearly enormous."

The adult negro brain is generally a little less than that of the white. Professor Tiedeman appears to deny this ; yet from his own examinations and admeasurements, it seems that the negro brain is something narrower in the anterior portion of the hemispheres than is usually the case in Europeans, that the average weight is less, the dimensions inferior and the average capacity of the skull not so large in the negro as in the European. The following table results from summing up his measurements of the cerebrum of negroes and whites.

		Inches.	Lines.
Average length of brain in	4 negroes	5	11
	7 European males	6	$2\frac{1}{7}$
	6 " females	5	$10\frac{1}{2}$
Average breadth of brain in	4 negroes	4	$8\frac{1}{2}$
	7 European males	5	$1\frac{1}{7}$
	3 " females	5	$4\frac{1}{3}$
Average height of brain in	3 negroes	2	$11\frac{1}{3}$
	7 European males	3	4
	4 " females	2	$9\frac{1}{2}$

I have weighed the brains of nine negroes none of which exceeded 3 lbs. 8 oz. In one instance of a large, well-formed negro, whose head was unusually large and

---

* Dictionnaire des Sciences Medicales, Vol. 22. Art. Hydrocephale. This statement of M. Itard, Physician to the Institution for the Deaf and Dumb at Paris, was written about the time of the abdication of Napoleon and is unquestionably correct.

well-developed, the skin was found uncommonly thick even for a negro, and the brain weighed 3 lbs. 8 oz. I was not able to learn any thing respecting his intellectual powers.

I have this day weighed the brain of a negro, apparently fifty years old, five feet ten and a half inches in height, large chest and head. The whole brain, including cerebrum and cerebellum, weighed 3 lbs. 6 oz. The cerebellum weighed a few grains less than 6 oz. I have not found the skull of the negro to be thicker than that of Europeans, but the scalp uniformly more so. But though the negro brain is usually a little smaller than that of Europeans, yet this difference may be owing to the greater amount of mental culture which the white race has for centuries received. In idiots the brain is usually small, varying, not uncommonly, in size with their intellectual powers. I have noticed that frequently there is no increase in the size of their heads after the age of eight or ten. Sometimes, however, their heads are of full size, or unnaturally large. In some instances the skull is much thicker than natural. The skull of an idiot, whose head was not badly formed, nor of unnatural size, who died in the Alms House of this city, was three quarters of an inch in thickness. The convolutions of the brain were small and compressed, and the whole brain quite diminutive.

The brain is divided into two portions, a superior and inferior, or the greater and lesser brain. The greater is called the cerebrum, the lesser the cerebellum. These are separated, to a considerable extent, by a thick strong membrane, stretched horizontally across from one side of the skull to the other, and which is but a fold of the dura mater, or of that membrane that lines the interior of the skull. The membrane which thus separates the greater from the lesser brain, is called the tentorium and serves to protect the lesser brain, the medulla oblongata and the upper part of the medulla spinalis from the weight of the upper or greater brain. Both the cerebrum and the cerebellum are divided into halves or hemispheres to a considerable extent. They are thus separated by a perpendicular fold of the dura mater called the falx, and which may serve to protect one side of the brain from the weight or concussion of the other. The external surface of the brain is convoluted or furrowed — that is, numerous clefts and divisions cut up apparently the outer portion of the brain into many irregular parts called convolutions. These convolutions covered by a thin membrane and net-work of blood-vessels, are all that we see on looking at the brain when the head is opened by removing the superior part of the skull, or when the brain is removed from the skull and placed on its base before us. On reversing the brain and looking at its base, or the under side of this organ we observe a a very different aspect. We notice *great irregularity* produced by the form of the skull and which gives occasion to divide the brain into an anterior, middle and posterior portion. We also now see the union of the greater and the lesser brain and their connection with the spinal marrow. The upper portion of the spinal marrow, or that which lies within the cranium, is seen much enlarged, and is called the medulla oblongata. At the upper part of the medulla oblongata is seen a large, thick, white band, nearly an inch in width, called the pons Varolii, and which unites the two portions of the cerebellum.

Above this band we also see two rounded fibrous bodies coming through the pons Varolii and diverging from each other into the hemispheres of the cerebrum. These are called the crura cerebri.

Having thus alluded to the external appearance of the brain we will now briefly notice some of the internal ar-

rangements of this organ. On cutting into, or cutting off
a portion of the brain, the first thing attracting attention is
the difference of color between the external and internal
parts of the brain. The outer part is of a grey color and
of a soft and pulpy texture, and appears to encircle the
inner, which is white and fibrous. The outer is called
the grey, the cineritous, or the cortical part of the brain ;
the inner is called the medullary, or white. The cineritious part envelopes all the convolutions, and by this arrangement — this folding up as it were, of the outer surface of the brain — its extent is greatly augmented beyond
what it would be if the surface was uniform and smooth.
This cineritious portion seems to receive a larger supply
of blood than the white, and while the latter is very similar in appearance and structure to the nerves, the cineritious bears no resemblance to any other part of the
system.

There are also some partial cavities called ventricles,
within the brain. There is a large one in each hemisphere of the cerebrum. These are called the lateral
ventricles, and are frequently found distended with fluid
after death from disease of the brain. On dissecting the
brain in various ways, parts have been seen which from
some resemblance to other objects, have received names
accordingly. These appearances and the names given
to them will be found in anatomical works, to which I refer the reader for more minute accounts of the structure
of the brain.*

On looking at the base of the brain we notice many
white cords or threads, apparently coming from the
brain, and in pairs, or one from each hemisphere. These
are called the cerebral nerves, and are numbered First,

---

* I would particularly recommend the work of Mr. Solly on "The
Human Brain, its Configuration, Structure," &c.   London, 1836.

Second, Third pairs, reckoning from the anterior to the posterior part of the brain. Some anatomists enumerate but nine pair of cerebral nerves, others eleven and twelve. This difference among authors respecting the number of the cerebral nerves, arises from some considering the seventh pair, consisting of the facial and auditory, as two pairs instead of one; and the glosso-pharyngeal and pneumo-gastric, which by some are called one pair, are by others divided into two. Some consider the spinal accessory as an associate of the pneumo-gastric and glosso-pharyngeal. I shall treat of twelve distinct pair of cerebral nerves. Viz:

1. Olfactory.
2. Optic.
3. Oculo-muscular.
4. Inner-oculo-muscular, or pathetic.
5. Trigeminal.
6. Abducentes.
7. Facial, or portio-dura.
8. Auditory, or portio-mollis.
9. Glosso-pharyngeal.
10. Pneumo-gastric, or par-vagum.
11. Lingual, or hyo-glossal.
12. Spinal-accessory.

These nerves are connected with the brain nearly at the same place ; in a small circle including the pons Varolii, medulla oblongata, corpora quadrigemina and a portion of the crura cerebri. But the point of connection of each nerve with the nervous mass within the cranium, so far as has been ascertained, will be pointed out when treating of the disease of these nerves.

The *medulla spinalis*, which appears like an appendage to the brain, to which it is connected by the medulla oblongata, is seen extending through the vertebral column or bony case, by which it is carefully protected. Con-

3

nected with the medulla spinalis are thirty-one pairs of nerves. Each of these nerves is attached to the spinal cord by two sets of filaments, or roots, called the anterior and the posterior roots of the spinal nerves.

Premising these few anatomical facts respecting the brain, the spinal marrow and the nerves, let us now proceed to ascertain what are the functions of these organs.

SECTION II.

FUNCTIONS OF THE BRAIN—METHODS ADOPTED FOR DETERMINING.

But how shall we proceed ? Is there any method by which we can determine the functions of the different parts of the brain ? If we were to judge from the vast labor and thought that have been bestowed upon this inquiry and consider how little has been ascertained, we might almost despair of succeeding by any further researches ; but when we call to mind that within a few years some new and important facts have been made known, far more than for centuries previous, we ought to be encouraged to continue our inquiries.

The methods resorted to for the purpose of determining the functions of the brain have been various, but I believe they may be noticed under the seven following heads.

1. Chemical analysis.
2. Dissection of the brain.
3. Experiments on living animals.
4. Comparative anatomy.

5. The fœtal condition and growth of the brain.
6. Pathological observations.
7. External examination of the cranium.

We will now examine these methods and learn how far each has contributed, or may be made to contribute, to extend our knowledge of the functions of the brain.

1. *Chemical analysis.* From the composition of some parts of the body we may perhaps infer something of their use. Thus we should know something of the use of the bones, the chyle and the blood, if we knew their component parts ; but nothing has been learned by analysing the brain that has added to our knowledge of its functions. It has, however, been carefully performed. M. John* is, I believe, the only chemist who has analysed separately the cineritious and the medullary portions The following comparative analysis was made by him of the brain of an insane person who died at Salpetriere.

	Entire brain, (density—1048.)	White substance.	Grey sub.
Water,	77.0	73.0	85.0
Albumen,	9.6	9.8	7.5
White fatty matter	7.2	13.9	1.0
Red fatty matter,	3.1	0.9	3.7
Osmazome, lactic acid and salts,	2.0	1.0	1.4
Earthy phosphate,	1.1	1.3	1.2

From this analysis it seems that the white portion of the brain contains more fatty matter than the grey, and he observes that its albumen is firmer. These differences may result, however, from disease, as it will be recollected that his analysis was of the brain of an insane patient.

Though I have said that the brain is composed of two substances, the grey and the white, yet there is a small

* Journal de Chimie Medicale, August, 1835.

portion of it, called the pineal gland, which has derived distinction from Descartes having considered it the seat of the soul, and which differs in composition from the other parts of the brain. This body situated near the base of the brain, usually contains some gritty matter. This has been analysed by M. Wurrer, of Marburg, and found to consist of carbonate and phosphate of lime, iron and manganese.

Though it is not probable that any important facts would be learned by further analysing the brain, yet it is to be desired that the different portions of the healthy brain of the new-born, the child, the adult, the aged and the male and the female, be analysed and compared.

2. *Dissection of the brain.* By dissecting and examining the structure of some parts of the system we may conjecture with considerable certainty their use. The examination of the heart and blood-vessels, for instance, would guide us considerably in our inquiries respecting their functions. But as relates to a knowledge of the functions of the brain, dissecting this organ affords us no light. We find by this method cavities and parts variously arranged and differing in color, but we learn nothing of their use. We may infer from the soft and delicate structure of the brain, that it cannot perform any of the functions of other organs ; and from its great size, its vast supply of blood, (according to the estimates of Malpighi and Haller, one third of the whole is sent to the brain,) and the extreme care with which it is protected by a bony envelopment, we may conclude its office is of great importance.

The difference in situation and appearance of the cerebrum and the cerebellum, the one much larger and placed above the other ; the greater having large and irregular convolutions, the lesser being lamellar, or having its folds lie in regular plates, affords good ground for supposing a difference of function, though anatomical examination and knowledge of the structure of the brain does not teach us what those functions are.

Again, the division of both the greater and lesser brain into halves deserves attention. It supports the opinion that whatever may be the functions of the brain, that each half is capable of executing them. An affection deeply seated in the brain sometimes destroys the sight of one eye, while the other is not affected. So we may not unreasonably suppose, from the double appearance of the brain, that its functions may be performed by either portion. So the difference in color and structure, noticed between the grey and white substance of the brain, leads us to infer, that their functions are different, as difference in structure indicates difference of function, yet the appearance of neither teaches us any of their uses.

The substance of the brain has been examined with great care by the aid of magnifying glasses. The most celebrated researches of this kind have been made by Sir Everard Home* and his coadjutor M. Bauer, and more recently by Professor Ehrenberg.† According to the microscopical observations of Sir E. Home and M. Bauer, the brain is composed of an elastic, transparent, viscid jelly, an aqueous albuminous fluid, blood-vessels and globules; that the globules are spherical and vary in size from $\frac{1}{2400}$ to $\frac{1}{4000}$ parts of an inch in diameter. They are of a semi-transparent white color, and arranged in threads or fibres of single globules, and apparently

---

* Sir Everard Home's two Croonian lectures read to the Royal Society in 1820 and 1823 and published in their Transactions.

† Observations on the Structure hitherto unknown of the Nervous System in Man and Animals. By Professor Ehrenberg, read to the Academy of Sciences in Berlin, in 1833, and published in the Transactions of the Berlin Academy in 1836.

3*

held together by the viscid mucus or jelly. These fibres form bundles connected in the same way. The cortical substance differs from the white, chiefly in the smaller size of its arteries and veins, and also by containing a yellow fluid resembling the serum of the blood.

The microscopical discoveries of Professor Ehrenberg are not only the most recent, as to the minute structure of the brain, but are considered altogether the most important. The glasses used by him had a magnifying power of 350 to 360 diameters, though he frequently employed, as means of testing the accuracy of his observations, glasses that magnified to the extent of 3000 diameters. But he found that glasses of the greatest attainable magnifying power rendered the inner figure less definite and clear.

Professor E. claims to have discovered in the brain and nervous system two sets of tubes, both hollow, the one presenting at short intervals globular expansions resembling a string of beads, these he calls varicose or *articulated* tubes and claims to have proved that they contain a peculiar matter which he calls *nervous fluid*. These are found chiefly in the brain, some in the spinal marrow and in the three soft nerves or those of proper sensation, the Olfactory, Optic and Auditory, but in none of the other nerves except in the middle of the great sympathetic.

Another set of tubes which are straight and uniform he calls *cylindrical*, they are larger than the articulated tubes and contain a viscid white, but rather turbid matter to which he has given the name of *medulla*. These cylindrical tubes are formed mostly in the nervous trunks and cords, but are not found in the nerves clearly devoted to sensation. He has however traced the cylindrical tubes of the motiferous nerves into the cortical substance, and found them continuations of the articulated tubes.

Hence he considers the nervous matter as well as the brain to consist everywhere of articulated tubules, conveying nervous fluid, and cylindrical tubules conveying true nervous medulla. He observes " the articulated nerve-tubes void of medulla according to their proportion of the human organism, and their distribution in the animal kingdom, constitutes the more important and noble part of the nervous system, ministering directly to sensation."

The cortical portion of the brain appears by his researches to differ from the medullary, by wanting for the most part, the cylindrical tubes, and having the articulated tubes contained in a thick vascular net-work. This part also contains a very fine grained soft substance, in which here and there are deposited larger grains in contact with the articulated tubes. This fine grained matter is confined to the grey portion of the convoluted surface of the brain. In concluding his researches Professor E. inquires, " Would not therefore, seemingly the nervous energies be a secretion from the blood of a material, and especially of these grains ; which first, in the form of a tough fluid, is collected in the articulated tubes, and gradually in that of nervous medulla is accumulated in the cylindrical tubes, advancing tardily and imperceptibly, till at their ends, it again, as excreted matter, passes into the general absorption. The distillation of the nervous *medulla* from the blood, appears then to be immediately the developement of that mysterious mental process which indicates itself, as sensation, and which, growing with the growth of the body, augments to complete consciousness. The circumstance, that man, by reason of the extent and the convoluted disposition of the largest surface of the brain, presents consequently the most extensive secretion of nervous fluid, may bear a direct relation to his mental energy."

Though these curious discoveries have been to some extent verified by others, yet the microscope has too often led us into error, to command now implicit confidence. It is however to be hoped that these researches will be continued, as they may yet serve to throw important light upon the functions of the nervous system, though we can hardly be permitted to say that they have yet done so.

3d. *Experiments on living animals.*

The method of determining the functions of the brain by vivisection has been resorted to by many Physiologists, especially by those on the continent of Europe, by Haller, Lorry, Finn, Rolando, Magendie, Serres, Fodere, Flourens, Bouillaud, and many others.

These distinguished Physiologists have seemed to suppose they might ascertain the functions of the brain by removing portions of this organ from living animals, and otherwise mutilating it, and noticing the effects produced. With this object in view they have tortured and killed innumerable animals, and I regret to say nothing important has been satisfactorily established by their sacrifice. Undoubtedly it is sometimes proper to have recourse to experiments on living animals, but it appears to me that such as torture and kill them, should not be resorted to without the advantages likely to result are obviously important. I cannot justify such procedure without any more definite object in view, than the mere hope that something may be learned by mutilating and torturing animals.

As respects the elucidation of the subject we are now discussing, experiments on animals cannot be of much avail. An insuperable objection in my mind is, that we cannot cut away a part of the brain without effecting the portion that remains, and of giving such a shock to the whole nervous system that but little can be inferred from the actions of animals after such operations. We know that very different sensations and symptoms follow from operations on men. One individual endures an operation without complaining, another complains greatly; one is scarcely effected in body or mind, another is prostrated as respects both. Go into the office of a Dentist and notice the conduct of those who have teeth extracted. One endures the operation without manifesting any disturbance of mind or body, another faints, another is convulsed, and another for a time is delirious. The lower animals, even those of the same species, differ as regards sensibility also. This every one conversant with them must have observed. One is extremely timid, easily affected, complaining bitterly of injuries, while another nothing can daunt, and no injury cause to complain. Some will remain quiet after operations, and move or eat reluctantly, while others appear active and eat readily.

Owing considerably if not chiefly to this difference in the sensibility of animals, we find that those who have performed similar experiments upon them, witnessed and described different results. Still I do not intend to say that no light has been thrown upon the physiology of the brain by these experiments, for some of them appear to me to be satisfactory to a considerable extent, and tend to confirm results obtained by other methods of investigation.

The most important experiments relating to the functions of the brain have been performed by Flourens, Bouillaud and Serres. M. Flourens' consisted principally in removing as far as he was able the part of the brain, the particular function of which he wished to ascertain.

" M. Flourens has pricked the *hemispheres* without producing either contractions of the muscles or any apparent pain to the animal ; he has removed them by slices. He has performed the same operation on the *cerebellum.* He has at the same time removed the hemisphere and the cerebellum ; the animal has remained impassive. The *corpora striata,* the *thalami nervorum opticorum* were attacked and removed without any effect. Contraction of the iris did not take place, neither was it paralysed.

" But when he irritated the *quadrigeminal tubercles,* shiverings and convulsions commenced ; and this shivering and these convulsions increased as he penetrated deeper into the medulla oblongata.

" The irritation of these tubercles as well as that of the optic nerves, produced violent and prolonged contractions of the iris."

" In his language, M. Flourens concludes that ' the medulla oblongata and quadrigeminal tubercles are irritable ;' which, in our language, signifies that they are conductors of irritation, as are the spinal marrow and nerves ; but that the cerebrum and cerebellum have not this property.

" The author also concludes that these tubercles are the continuation and termination of the spinal marrow and medulla oblongata ; and this conclusion is in accordance with what their anatomical relations and connexions indicate."

" After the effects of ablation of the brain, properly so called, M. Flourens examines those of the extirpation of the quadrigeminal tubercles. The removal of one of the two, after a convulsive action which immediately ceases, produces blindness of the opposite eye, and an involuntary whirling round ; that of the two tubercles renders the cecity complete and the whirling more violent and more prolonged. Yet the animal retains all its faculties, and the iris is still contractile. The entire extirpation, or a section of the optic nerve alone, paralyses the iris; from which circumstance M. Flourens concludes that extirpation of the tubercle produces the same results as a section of the nerve ; that this tubercle is as regards vision only a conductor ; and that the cerebral lobe alone is the limit of the sensation, and the place where it is consummated by becoming converted into perception. After all it must be observed that in too deeply extirpating these tubercles we interfere with the medulla oblongata, and then violent convulsions, which last long, make their appearance. What appears to us to be most curious and unheard of in M. Flourens' experiments, concerns the functions of the cerebellum. During the ablation of the first slices, only a little weakness and a want of harmony in the movements occur. At the removal of the middle slices an almost general agitation is the result. The animal, continuing to hear and to see, only executes abrupt and disorderly movements. Its faculties of flying, walking, standing up, &c. are lost by degrees. When the cerebellum is removed, the faculty of performing regulated movements has entirely disappeared. Placed on its back the creature could not get up ; yet it saw the blow that threatened it, it heard noises, it endeavored to avoid danger, and made many efforts to do so without accomplishing its object. In a few words, it retained the faculties of perception and of volition, but it had lost the power of making its muscles obey its will. It was with difficulty that a bird stood up, resting upon its wings and tail. Deprived of its brain, it was in a dormant state ; deprived of its cerebellum, it was in a state of apparent drunkenness."*

---

* Report made to the Royal Academy of Sciences of the Institute on the Memorial of M. Flourens, 1822.

M. Bouillaud* repeated these experiments and came to nearly the same conclusions, though he believes the regulating power of the cerebellum extends only to the muscles of locomotion. " Mutilations of the cerebellum," says he, " were not accompanied by paralysis or convulsions, properly so called, but merely by disorder of the locomotive functions ; the faculties of equilibrium and progression were destroyed. The animals mutilated were still capable of reflection, of hearing, of moving their limbs in all directions, and most frequently these movements were executed with extraordinary quickness and violence ; from which it follows," says M. Bouillaud, " that we must admit the existence in the cerebellum of a force which presides over the association of the movements composing the different acts of locomotion and of station, a force essentially distinct from that which governs the simple movements both of the trunk and limbs, although there exists the most intimate connection between the two.

" In this view of the subject it is impossible not to adopt the opinion of M. Flourens, namely, that in the cerebellum resides the power of co-ordinating the actions of walking, running, flying, standing, &c. But M. Flourens appears to have fallen into an error when he says, that the cerebellum is the co-ordinator of all the movements called voluntary.

" Up to this time experiments only warrant our saying that the cerebellum is the central nervous organ which gives to vertebrated animals the faculty of preserving their equilibrium and of exercising the various acts of locomotion."

---

*"Recherches Cliniques et Experimentales tendant a refuter l'opinion de M. Gall sur les Fonctions du Cervelet, et a prouver que cet organe preside aux actes de l'Equilibration, de la Station et de la Progression."

M. Foville* admits these facts, but thinks they prove that the cerebellum is the central seat of sensibility, that it is because sensibility is destroyed, because the animal does not feel the ground it treads upon, nor the objects it runs against, nor is sensible of its own muscular movements, that it fails to keep its equilibrium.

" The opinion advanced by some physiologists," says M. Foville, " that the cerebellum is the regulator of the voluntary movements, if we attentively consider the reasoning on which it rests, seems to me to strengthen the idea which places the central seat of sensibility in the cerebellum. After having injured the structure of the cerebellum extensively, we have observed that animals preserved the power of moving their limbs, but had lost that of co-ordinating the movements of these in a manner convenient to station, progression, flight, &c. But when we *will* to perform, and actually perform, certain movements, do we not distinctly feel that we execute them ? The man who, with his eyes shut, moves his hand or his arm, does he not also as distinctly feel that he moves these parts as if he followed them with his eyes ? whilst the paralysed man who, with his eyes shut, is desired to move the paralysed limbs, may be very willing to do so, though incapable, and perfectly aware of his incapability of obeying ; nor would it be possible to persuade the individual so circumstanced that he did move his limbs.

" If this be true, (and no one, I think, will doubt it,) how can we expect that an animal deprived of the faculty of perceiving the sensation of the movements which it executes should execute them in the *ensemble* with harmony and in accordance with a proposed end ? How

---

* Dictionnaire de Medicine et de Chirurgie Pratique, Vol. 7th, Art. Encephale, p. 204.

can we expect it to walk deliberately and keep its equilibrium, if it does not feel the ground upon which it stands, if it is ignorant of the position in which its limbs are placed ?   Sir Astley Cooper with whom I conversed on this subject towards the end of the year 1830, cited to me the case of a man completely deprived of the faculty of sensation in one arm and hand, the muscular power of which was, however, preserved.   When this man was desired to take hold of and to lift anything, he did so very well; but if, whilst holding the object, his attention was taken away from the hand, irregular contractions of the limb commenced, and very soon the object held fell to the ground: as soon as the patient ceased to follow the contractions of his fingers with his eyes, nothing remained to inform him that he held the object, when, of course, it escaped from his grasp."

M. Serres, from some experiments and cases, is of the opinion that the cerebellum, especially its median lobe, is the exciter of the genital organs.   He says, " Oxen knocked down by a blow in the occiput, which tears the cerebellum, have the penis considerably affected ;" and states that a stallion manifested decided erection, when a knife was plunged into the median lobe of the cerebellum.   M. Segalas, induced erection in a guinea pig, by plunging a knife deep into the cerebellum, so as to arrive at the upper part of the spinal marrow.   Other experimenters have obtained somewhat different results.   Magendie found that a duck would only swim backward after the cerebellum was removed, and that if the right crus of the cerebellum was cut through, the animal whirled round incessantly, from left to right, for twenty-four hours.   If both were divided no movement occurred. Fodere found that the removal of a part of the cerebellum was followed by motion backward.

If we admit the correctness of the results alluded

to from these experiments, they teach us but little. About all that we may infer from them, is, that the hemispheres of the cerebrum are the seat of consciousness, of memory, and the intellectual faculties, and that the cerebellum is connected with the locomotive powers and the function of generation, and essential to their healthful and orderly manifestation. It is well known that Gall located the function of generation in the cerebellum, but supposed it might have other. "We should never forget," says he, " that one and the same part may have its general vital function, and its particular animal function besides. The cerebellum may participate in the vital function of the medulla spinalis and medulla oblongata, and, at the same time, have a particular animal function."*

We must therefore have recourse to other methods of investigation than those of vivisection, to satisfy ourselves respecting the functions of the brain.

4. *Comparative Anatomy.* — Examining the brain of the lower animals, and comparing them with those of man, in connection with the mental powers manifested, has been resorted to by some with the view of ascertaining the functions of the human brain. This method can be of no avail only for a part of the mental faculties, as man exhibits many that other orders of animals do not. But the examination and comparison so far as it has been carried, satisfactorily shows this increased development of the brain is always accompanied by increased mental power.

The animal kingdom, like to the vegetable and the mineral, has been divided by naturalists into sub-king-doms, classes, orders, &c. The arrangement of Cuvier,

---

* On the Functions of the Brain and each of its parts, &c. Boston edition Gall's Works, Vol. 3d, p. 244–5.

though not founded on any fixed principles, has been generally adopted.   These sub-kingdoms are,

1. Radiated.
2. Articulated.
3. Molluscous.
4. Vertebrated.

Other naturalists considering the superior importance of the nervous system, have sought to establish the grand divisions of the animal kingdom in its modifications. Lamark proposed three great divisions founded on the intellectual manifestations of animals — Apathic, or Automatic, the Sensitive, and the Intelligent.

Professor Grant, of the London University, has made divisions which though founded upon the differences in the nervous system, corresponds to the divisions of Cuvier, as follows :

1. Cyclo-neurose of Grant is   Radiated of Cuvier.
2. Diplo-neurose   Articulated.
3. Cyclo-gangliated   Molluscous.
4. Spini-cerebrata   Vertebrated.

1st. In the lowest class of animals, the *Radiated*, we do not always find the nervous system sufficiently distinct to be demonstrated.   Whenever it is perceptible, it is found in delicate circular filaments about the mouth. Founded upon this condition of the nervous system the name of Cyclo-neurose has been given to this class of animals.   The Porifera, or sponges, Asterias, or star-fish, and Physalia, the Portuguese man of war, are of this division.

2d. The *Articulated* of Cuvier, and Diplo-neurose of Grant, including the tape-worm, earth-worm, leech, lobster, spider and insects, are endowed with a more extended nervous system, consisting of a double nervous cord, or column extending along the whole vertebral surface of the body.

3d. The *Molluscous* of Cuvier is the Cyclo-gangliated of Grant, and has the nervous system more abundant in the vascular, digestive, and glandular apparatus, and more concentrated around the entrance of the alimentary canal, where it generally forms transverse series of ganglia, disposed around the œsophagus, thence the term Cyclo-gangliated. The snail and the oyster are examples of this division of animals.

4th. *Vertebrata* of Cuvier. The Spini-cerebrata of Grant, have a lengthened dorsal, nervous cord, developed anteriorly into a brain, and protected by a vertebral column and cranium. In this division are classed the Fishes, Amphibia, Reptiles and the Mammalia.

Thus it will be seen that the *First* primary division of animals is but slightly endowed with a nervous system, a few filaments around the mouth to endow them with taste or feeling, and enabling them to reject or receive whatever presents itself at the mouth.

The *Second* division has a larger nervous system, one that extends down the anterior part of the body. The *Third* has a still larger, and it is more concentrated around the alimentary organs, giving more perfection to the digestive, circulatory, and glandular system. Some of them have ganglia so large and concentrated as to nearly entitle them to the name of brain; in fact the brain of the higher order of animals appears to be a collection and concentration of ganglia. The *Fourth* division is characterized by a far superior nervous system, consisting of a nervous cord protected by the vertebral column and expanded into more or less of a brain protected by a cranium.

But if we direct our attention to this last division, the Vertebrata, we find many marked differences in the nervous system, especially in the formation of the brain of the animals of the different classes into which it has been

4*

subdivided, viz : Fishes, Amphibia, Reptiles, Birds and Mammalia.

In *Fishes* — we find the spinal portion of the nervous system very similar to that of man ; the nerves arise from it by anterior and posterior filaments, the posterior having a small ganglion connected with them, the same as in man. But the brain in fishes scarcely deserves the name, as it is but a slight enlargement of the spinal cord. About $\frac{1}{30}$ is the average proportion of the weight of the brain to the body of an adult man, while in a fish the weight of the body, in comparison with the human brain, predominates immensely. The brain of the shark, for instance, is but as *one* to two thousand four hundred and ninety-six, compared with the weight of its body. Still the rudiments of the hemispheres, or lobes of the cerebrum, and a structure corresponding to the cerebellum, though small, may be distinguished, and these superior nervous endowments undoubtedly confer upon them higher intellectual powers, such as memory, than are possessed by animals belonging to the inferior divisions. In the nervous system of the Amphibia, or vertebrated animals with cold blood, and most of them undergoing a metamorphosis, or change of condition, having relation to a transition from an aquatic to an atmospheric medium of respiration, we find the condition of the brain in their early or pisiform state very similar to that of Fishes. But when they pass into the Reptile state the brain receives additional development in a very short time — the hemispheres become enlarged laterally and superiorly, and they now manifest higher intellectual powers than before their metamorphosis.

The nervous system of Reptiles is very similar to that of the Amphibia after they have passed from their early and imperfect condition ; and by many the Amphibia are considered not a distinct class, but an order of Reptiles.

Birds. — The nervous system of Birds is developed to a much higher degree than that of any class of animals we have alluded to. " The brain of the bird differs from that of the reptile in the superior size of the cerebrum, and the more complex structure of the cerebellum. It differs from the brain of a mammal in the smaller size of the cerebellum, resulting from the want of the lateral lobes, and in the absence or rudimentary condition of the fornix ; and it differs from the brain of every other vertebrated class, in the lateral and inferior position of the optic lobes, or bigeminal bodies."*

The superior size of the cerebral lobes of birds corresponds to their advance in intellect on the other classes mentioned, still these lobes present a smooth surface, as they are without convolutions which we find in the higher order of animals, the mammalia, and by which arrangement the cineritious neurine is much increased.

Mammalia. — " The advance which the brain makes in this class of animals is very striking. The spinal cord no longer competes with it in point of dimensions. The hemispheres, except in the very lowest members of the class, begin to take on a convoluted appearance, and the optic tubercles, instead of remaining merely a single pair, have, appended to their posterior surface, two additional and smaller masses of medullary neurine, called the testes. But still we do not find any sudden transition from one form of brain to another ; there is no great chasm between the brain in Birds and that of the Mammalia, for when we direct our attention to the brain of the Rodentia, or gnawing animals, we find almost as much difference between its anatomy in them and in man, as between that of the feathered race and the lord of the creation. The upper surface of the hemi-

---

* R. Owen, Esq. Cyclopedia of Anatomy and Physiology.

spheres in the rat, mouse, marmot, beaver, and even in the rabbit, is as smooth as in birds ; the hemispheres in most of these animals do not cover the cerebellum, and in some instances not even the optic tubercles."

Among this large class of animals we observe great disparity of intellect, but uniformly find an increase of brain accompanying the manifestation of superior intellect. Those animals that nearest approach man in regard to mental powers, as the ourang-outang, have a brain bearing a closer resemblance to that of man than other animals. For a striking instance of this connection between cerebral development and mental power I need but refer to the anatomical structure of the brain of the Porpoise.

" This creature, which to the vulgar is no more than a large fish, the enlightened physiologist admits into the same grand division of the animal kingdom to which man himself belongs. Bringing forth its young in a state requiring long after birth the protecting care of the mother, higher moral and intellectual endowment are implied than we can expect in fishes and reptiles, whose spawn is generally abandoned by the parent as soon as it is shed ; and in accordance with these manifestations of higher powers, we find the cerebral mass developed upon the same plan and presenting nearly the same appearances and arrangement of parts as some of the most perfect of the terrestrial mammalia, and even as the brain of man himself."

But from the examination of the brain of animals, comparing them with that of man, and watching their mental manifestations, about all we learn is that enlargement of the brain, especially of the anterior and superior portions, is ever accompanied by an augmentation of mental power. In many of the lower animals the base of the brain and the spinal marrow differs but little from that of man.

It is therefore not unreasonable to conclude that the upper or superior part of the brain, which man possesses, and which other animals do not, enables him to exhibit superior mental powers.

It may be proper here to notice some other methods resorted to for ascertaining the mental capacity of the different classes of animals. One is by considering the *size* of the brain as the sole evidence of mental power, and then comparing the brains of different animals.

But it has been proved, that if this was true man should have inferior intellect to the elephant and whale, both of which have brains larger than that of man. Again it was said man had the largest brain in proportion to the size of his body, but this was found not to be correct, as some monkeys, the canary bird, &c., have larger brains in proportion to the size of their bodies than man.

Others said that the brain of man in comparison to the size of the spinal marrow was larger than in any other animal, and this accounted for his superior powers of mind. But this according to Cuvier is not a fact, as the Dolphin and some other animals are exceptions.

Let us here briefly allude to the celebrated "*facial angle*," of Camper, which may be considered another method of determining the intellectual powers, and which consists in comparing the brain with the size of the bones of the face. This angle is formed by a line drawn horizontally from the roots of the incisor teeth of the upper jaw to the meatus externus, and then intersected by a line drawn perpendicularly from the same point at the teeth to the most elevated point of the forehead. Of course the more the forehead projects, the greater will be the angle, hence when the anterior lobes of the brain are greatly developed, the angle is increased. There is to be sure some little truth in this method of comparison,

But as a guide to determine the difference of the mental powers it is very defective. The facial angle of the infant is generally greater than that of the adult, and in the most stupid of the white race superior to that of the most intelligent of negroes; and besides, in three quarters of the animals of various degrees of intelligence, says Blumenbach, the facial angle is the same.

5. *The fœtal condition and growth of the Brain.*

This is perhaps, entitled to be considered another method of determining the functions of the brain. It consists in watching the early developement and growth of the brain and marking the mental manifestations at different stages. This study is most curious and interesting, though perhaps of little utility in relation to the subject we are investigating. Meckel, Tiedemann, Serres, Geoffroy St. Hiliare and others have examined the growth of the fœtal brain with great attention, and their observations are exceedingly curious. According to these authorities the brain of the human fœtus in the earliest months of its existence resembles that of some of the lower order of animals; when a few months older it receives additional parts, which cause it to resemble that which animals of a higher order always retain; but that it is not until the time of birth or afterwards that parts are added which distinguish it from the brain of other animals. The most important conclusions which may be drawn from these investigations are thus summed up by Mr. Anderson.* " Nature follows an uniform plan in the creation and evolution both of the brain of the human fœtus and that of vertebral animals.

---

* Sketch of the Comparative Anatomy of the Nervous System, with remarks on its developement in the human embryo. By John Anderson, London, 1837.

The brain of the human fœtus, at certain stated periods during its passage from a simple to a complicated state, is twice represented in nature; that is, by a permanent form, and by a transient form of the brain of a lower class of animals. Thus, the human fœtal brain at the fourth month, is permanently represented by the reptiles, and transiently represented by the fœtal chick at the sixteenth day, and the fœtal sheep at the eighth week.

The analogies in the structure of the brain in the human fœtus, and in animals, are uniform in their existence, and are applicable to each portion of the cerebral mass, at one stated period of its developement in man, and in one particular class of animals. Thus, the analogy in the conformation of the human fœtal brain, at the fourth month, and in the reptiles, exists in each portion of cerebral mass, and not in one particular portion only.

The definite periods at which these analogies are most apparent may be established as follows—

Humun Fœtal Brain.	*Brain of Animals.*
3d month,	Fishes,
4th month,	Reptiles,
5th month,	Birds,
6th month,	Mammalia (Ruminatia, Carnivora,) &c.
7th month,	Mammalia (Lower Quadrumana)
8th month,	Mammalia, (Highest Quadrumana,")

Sometimes this process of fœtal developement is arrested in some of the organs and then a being is born, exhibiting as to the organ affected an arrangement similar to that permanently retained by inferior animals. Thus we may account for certain monstrosities. But these and similar investigations though exceedingly interesting and deserving of profound attention, teach us but little more respecting the functions of the brain than what we have already learned, that mental power is in proportion to cerebral developement, especially of the anterior and superior portions of the cerebral lobes.

6. *Pathological Observations.*

Let us now direct our attention to one other method of investigating the functions of the brain, a method which as I have already intimated, we shall be richly re-paid for pursuing.   The method I allude to, is that of Pathological investigation — to careful dissection of the brain of those who have died from affections of this or-gan, and noticing the symptoms manifested during life. Sir Everard Home, some years since directed the atten-tion of medical men to this manner of investigating this subject.   " The various attempts," says he, " which have been made to procure accurate information respecting the functions that belong to individual portions of the human brain, having been attended with very little suc-cess, it has occurred to me, that were anatomical sur-geons to collect, in one view, all the appearances they had met with, in case of injury of that organ, and of the effects that such injuries produced upon its functions, a body of evidence might be formed, that would materially advance this highly important investigation."*

We have already learned something of importance by this method of investigating the subject.

First, we have, it appears to me, ascertained from Pathological observations that the functions of the ciner-itious and the medullary portions of the brain are quite different — that the cineritious portion of the brain is more particularly concerned in intellectual operations, while the office of the medullary part is to conduct sen-

---

* Philosophical Transactions, for 1814.

sation and volition; that when the medullary part is
alone affected, disturbance of motion occurs, but not of
the intellect, and that when the cineritious portion is diseased, the intellect is alone affected. The following
statements tend to establish these views.

In the writings of medical men we find numerous cases
of delirium arising from inflammation which is confined
principally to the membranes of the brain. These membranes surely have nothing to do with the manifestations of
intellect, but the disease which affects them, extends to
the cortical substance of the brain, and thus occasions
derangement of the mind.

"The fact of delirium occurring so frequently in inflammation of the membranes of the brain, is of considerable
importance, as showing, not that membranes of the brain
have any thing to do with intelligence, but as supporting
the opinions of those who believe the periphery of the
brain to be the seat of the intellectual faculties, and here
is a fact, which, as far as it goes, is in favor of the doc-
trines of phrenology. If we compare those cases of cerebral disease in which there is delirium, with those in
which it does not occur, we shall find that it is most common in cases where disease attacks the periphery of the
brain, as in arichnitis. The cases in which we observe
great lesions of the brain without delirium, are generally
cases of deep-seated inflammations of a local nature, or inflammation of those portions of the brain which the phrenologists consider not to be subservient to the production
of mental phenomena. This fact, also, would seem to confirm the truth of the opinion of the difference in function
between the medullary and cortical parts of the brain.
It is supposed that the cortical part of the brain is the
organ of intelligence, while the medullary portion per-
forms a different function. It is, however, a curious fact
that in delirium the inflammation is generally confined to

5

the surface of the brain, and that in cases of deep-seated inflammation, the most important symptoms are those which are derived from the sympathetic affections of the muscular system."*

From the manner in which the membranes of the brain and the contiguous cerebral substance are supplied with blood, both from the same source, it is evident that the one could not be much inflamed, and the other remain unaffected. " It is impossible," says Lallemand, " that the arachnoid should be inflamed without the surface of the brain in contact with it being also affected ; but its tissue not being altered, there merely results from this vicinity, exaltation in its functions." This makes it exceedingly difficult if not impossible to say with certainty what symptoms indicate inflammation of the one and not of the other. "Our knowledge of the subject," says Abercrombie,† " is not sufficiently matured to enable us to say with confidence what symptoms indicate inflammation of the substance of the brain, as distinguished from inflammation of its membranes."

M. M. Bayle, Martinet, and others, have published cases of what they call Arachnitis, for the purpose of establishing the diagnosis and pathology of Inflammation of the Arachnoid Membrane. But on examining these cases we find most of them presented marks of the inflammation having extended to the cerebral substance, the vessels of the pia mater being injected and the external surface of the brain exhibiting abundant proof of having participated in the disease.

But as such cases do not present any deep-seated affection of the brain, as the medullary portion is not

---

* Dr. Stokes Lectures on Cerebral Diseases.

† Pathological and Practical researches on Diseases of the Brain and the Spinal cord.

altered, they may be properly referred to as evidencing that the cortical substance of the brain is the seat of intelligence.

It has also been noticed that inflammation of the membranes covering the convexity of the brain is accompanied with early and violent delirium, but that in inflammation of the membrane at the base of the brain on the peduncles and pons Varolii, the symptoms are more insidious, attended with convulsions and coma and often without delirium. Dr. Stokes referring to this subject observes, " According to the researches of some celebrated French pathologists, there are a number of facts to show that there is a remarkable difference between the symptoms of arachnitis of the convexity and of the base of the brain. This conclusion, which after a most careful series of investigations was adopted by them, is borne out by the results of my experience, and appears to me to be established on the basis of truth. They have discovered that arachnitis of the convexity of the brain is a disease characterized by prominent and violent symptoms, early and marked delirium, pain, and sleep-lessness, and then coma. But in arachnitis of the base of the brain, the symptoms are of a more latent and insidious character ; there is some pain, and the coma is profound, but there is often no delirium."

Cases illustrative of these facts are to be found in several authors. The two first are from Andral.*

CASE I. — A postillion, thirty-three years of age, of strong constitution, received, on the 2d February, 1822, on the right side of the neck, a very heavy sack of oats, which fell on him from the height of several feet. He,

* Clinique Medicale, or Reports of Medical Cases, by G. Andral. Translated by D. Spillan, M. D.

however, continued his customary occupation till the
7th. He felt a painful tension on the right side of the
neck, at which part the skin assumed an erysipelatous
appearance ; fever came on, and the patient kept his
room. The fever continued on the 8th, 9th, and 10th,
and the erysipelas spread. On the 11th he entered the
hospital, when the fever was very high ; the neck was
covered with leeches. Desquamation commenced at
several points of the skin of the neck ; but on the right,
behind the sterno-mastoid muscle, an obscure fluctuation
was observed ; this muscle also seemed more prominent
than that of the opposite side ; no other morbid symptom ;
no stool for three days. At one o'clock in the morning
the patient suddenly became delirious. On the 12th, at
eight o'clock, the delirium still continued ; eyes haggard,
constantly rolling ; pupils very much contracted ; violent
screams ; free motion of the limbs ; pulse frequent and
very weak ; tongue moist and red ; burning thirst ; no
stool ; some leeches applied the preceding day, still
bleeding ; (blister to one thigh, sinapisms to the legs,
purging enema, acid drink.) Three hours after the
visit he expired.

Post mortem. — Arachnoid and pia mater natural in
every respect, except for the space of three fingers
breadth in length and two in width, near the anterior
extremity of the upper surface of the left hemisphere of
the brain. There the membranes were thick and red.
A small quantity of limpid serum in each lateral ventricle ; the posterior part of the two lungs infarcted ; the
mucous membrane of the stomach presented, at the
pyloric portion, a slight brownish tint ; the spleen very
soft ; a great quantity of pus infiltrated the cellular tissue
beneath the sterno-mastoid muscle of the right side.

Remarks. — This is a very remarkable case. It is
probable that the partial arachnitis, ascertained in the

dead body, commenced only with the delirium; the disturbance of the intellect, and a striking contraction of the pupils, were the only two phenomena occasioned by this inflammation; at times these very slight inflammations of the meninges are sufficient to disturb the intellect. We may note also, that here the inflammation was seated at the anterior and superior part of one of the cerebral hemispheres, where, in fact, several physiologists more particularly place the seat of intellect.

Compare with this.

CASE II. — A laboring man, of middle age and strong constitution, on entering the hospital complained of nothing but a violent headache, which commenced five or six days previous, and was for the first two days accompanied with a painful vomiting. The temples were the seat of the pain; they seemed as if compressed in a vice; at intervals he felt acute lancinating pains either at the temple, or the occiput; and occasionally the back of the neck became so painful that the patient could not move: he then presented all the symptoms of wry neck — he felt easy only when perfectly at rest; appetite gone; and what he ate, he said, gave him no strength; since the invasion of the headache had been but once at stool. We saw him first on the 3d of July, when he presented the following state; — Face pale and dejected; look quite vacant; eyes very sensible to strong light; intellect clear; pulse and skin natural. The head-ache the only important symptom in this case; (bleeding to sixteen ounces; sinapisms to legs; purging clyster;) the blood formed in a soft coagulum, with little serum and no buff. 4th July. He complained aloud of the violent pain of his head; he fancied his skull beaten in as it were with a hammer. Still his forehead was cool, and his face paler than the day before,

5*

the pupils, INTELLECT, circulation, natural. Thus the
bleeding produced no diminution of the headache — (a
second bleeding.)   On the 5th thirty leeches were
applied to the neck.   On the 6th headache less ; but he
answered questions with difficulty ; he lies on his back
and remains motionless, and resembles a person going to
sleep, or whose eyelids are struggling against sleep.
He still retains his intellect, but appears to use it in spite
of himself ; countenance very pale ; features drawn, and
as it were fatigued.   (Two blisters to the legs.)   On the
7th he appears in a profound sleep, will not answer
questions ; when bid he puts out his tongue readily,
which remains white and moist.   On being pinched he
shows that he still retains all his sensibility ; pupils
sensible to light ; pulse sixty ; heat of skin natural.   8th
and 9th.   Profound coma ; he refuses to open his eyes,
and appears not to hear the questions put to him ; pupils
natural ; some sensibility still retained ; (strong sinapisms
to the lower extremities.)   On the 10th.   Coma still ;
complete loss of sensibility ; yet, notwithstanding this
annihilation of the functions of the life of relation, described
by the ancients under the name of lethargy, the functions
of organic life are still perfect ; pulse, temperature of
skin, and respiration natural.   On the 12th, for the first
time, the respiration appeared affected ; sometimes very
much accelerated, at other times so slow that the
respiratory movement just made, seemed not likely to
be succeeded by another.   On the 13th.   Respiration
still accelerated ; in the course of the day the tracheal
rattle set in, and the patient died in the night.

Post mortem. — The upper part of the brain and
meninges being minutely examined, no morbid appearance
was detected ; but on examining the lower surface, the
pia mater covering it was infiltrated with a purulent
layer from seven to eight lines thick.

The following from the conjoint work of Parent Duchatelet and Martinet,* is an interesting case, though the treatment appears to have been very inefficient.

CASE III. — Depurs, three and a half years of age, after enjoying good health, was taken on the 14th July, 1817, with spontaneous vomiting of greenish matter, which continued more or less until the 24th of the same month, accompanied with prostration of strength, a slight degree of drowsiness, and smart paroxysms of fever without delirium or restlessness. During all this time there was obstinate constipation and violent headache. The child frequently screamed out, and there were some convulsive movements about the eyes. The intellect did not seem disturbed. He was transported to the Hospital des Infans, on this day, the 11th of the disease, and the following symptoms were noted. The child lay on his back, the trunk immobile, head turned backwards, eyelids heavy and closed, pupils little dilated, features altered, eyes turned upwards. The child was sensible when spoken to, and complained of great pain in the occipital region — drowsiness constant, pulse feeble, irregular, and frequent; respiration slow, unequal and apparently difficult; tongue coated yellow; constipation. Mustard pediluvia, lavements, lemonade, nitric ether mixture. In two hours some convulsive movements, screaming, complains of violent pain in the back of the head, to which part the child was constantly applying his hand. Twelfth day, (second in hospital.) Piercing cries during the whole night; strabismus; features greatly altered. Lemonade with a grain of emetic tartar, lavements,

---

* Recherches sur l'Inflammation de l'Arachnoide, Cerebrale, et Spinale; ou Histoire Theorique et Pratique de l'Arachnitis. Paris. 1821.

mustard pediluvia; blister to the nape of the neck and behind the ears; ice to the head. In two hours a strong paroxysm; much crying during the day; loss of intellectual and sentient faculties. Thirteenth day, a general remission of all the symptoms; pulse very irregular; great irritability of temper. Same treatment. Fourteenth day, (third stage of the disease,) pupils dilated and immoveable; profound somnolency; pulse irregular, feeble, small and extremely quick; eyes prominent, affected with strabismus, and half open; head inclining to any position which the laws of gravity dictated; *the intellect not much affected.* Blisters to vertebral column. Fifteenth day, same state, but the intellect more disturbed. Sixteenth day, profound coma; gradual extinction of the vital and natural functions; death.

Dissection. — Arachnoid inflammation at the base of the brain, about the decussation of the optic nerves, and over the tuber annulare; the membrane itself covered, in many places, with an albuminous exudation, penetrating into the fissura magna sylvii. Eight ounces of serous effusion in the ventricles. No other morbid appearance in any part of the body.

The researches of M. Foville,* respecting the state of the brain in cases of insanity, have thrown considerable light on this subject. Few men have enjoyed so good opportunities for investigating diseases of the brain as M. Foville. In conjunction with his friends Delaye and P. Grandchamp, he carried on his inquiries for a considerable time at the great Hospital of the Salpetriere, when it was under the superintendence of M. Esquirol, and more recently at the extensive Hospital for the Insane at St. Yon, in the department of the Lower

---

* Dictionnaire de Med. and Chirurg. Prat. Vol. 1. Art. Alienation Mentale.

Seine, which for several years has been under his superintendence. His observations are entitled to the greater
weight, from his having adopted the judicious practice
of examining at the same time the brain of one who died
without any disease of this organ, and the brain of one
who died insane.

In acute cases of insanity he found the cineritious
portion of the brain, particularly the anterior part of the
cerebral lobes, intensely red, but without adhering to the
membranes. But in chronic cases he found the cortical
substance indurated and adherent to the membranes.
In some instances, in cases of long standing, he found the
convolutions lessened. He has also found the white
portion of the brain injected and hardened, and he
conceives that the fibres of the medullary substance have
in chronic cases contracted adhesions to each other. In
nearly all cases of insanity accompanied with general
paralysis he has noticed these adhesions and has also
observed hardness of the medullary substance. Similar
appearances he has also found in the brains of aged men
whose voluntary motions had become impaired.

M. Foville refers to the opinion advanced by M.
Calmiel, that paralysis occurring in the insane, was
connected with disease of the cineritious substance of the
brain. This he has shown to be incorrect by reference
to numerous cases of alteration of the cineritious portion,
without the least affection of movement. " I might
speak," he says, " of the many hundreds of observations
of this sort which I have made myself, or with my
colleagues Delaye and P. Grandchamp, and in which
marked alterations of the cortical substance of the brain
were not connected with any other phenomenon than
disorder of the intellect."

Cases in corroboration of these opinions of M. Foville
have been furnished by other writers. The following
remarks and cases from Bouillaud are to the purpose.

"If we reflect that disturbance of the intellect can exist independently of every other derangement of the cerebral functions, if we reflect moreover that disturbance of the intellect appears to coincide constantly with an alteration of the cortical substance of the brain, we shall be obliged to admit as very probable this double opinion, namely, that the injury of the intellect depends upon that of a distinct part of the cerebral mass, and that the distinct part of the brain the injury of which produces derangement of the intellect is the cortical substance of that organ."

CASE IV.— Maintion, 43 years of age, house-painter, married, entered the 18th of November, 1823, the hospital of La Charite: six years ago he left the military service, and had only been in Paris two months. Since two years he had shown signs of imbecility, and had completely lost all memory. Whilst he was a military man, he had shown at different periods derangement of the intellectual faculties. Last year, at Versailles, he had symptoms of acute meningitis: two months ago, these same symptoms having re-appeared, a seton was inserted in the nape of the neck: besides, for two years he has complained of constant pain of the head and at the root of the nose, with a smell of putrefaction in this cavity. For a twelvemonth *he has been weak in his legs.* He has always had a good appetite. After having taken cold-baths for a month when he was in the hospital of St. Michel, he fell in a state of great exhaustion, and experienced lypothymiæ.

" The 17th of November he lost his mind, had repeated attacks of convulsions, with loud and unequal respiration. The 18th, at ten in the morning, general convulsions; eyes wandering; white froth from the mouth; rigidity of the limbs; sometimes grinding of the teeth and contortion of the mouth; sensibility remaining in the upper extremities, which he draws back when pinched, and makes grimaces; no motion in the lower extremities when pinched, but they are less rigid than the upper. Total loss of intelligence; respiration rattling; pulse pretty strong, full, regular and slow. (*Thirty leeches to the neck, ice to the head, sinapisms to the inferior extremities, a purgative enema.*) The agitation continued the remainder of the day; the convulsions are universal; the face is red and tumefied, the mouth is deformed, the lips projecting anteriorly. With the ice, the head is exceedingly hot; the fore-arms are strongly flexed; intellect is entirely lost. He was in the same state during the night. The 19th, in the morning, the right arm is almost without motion, the left alternately rigid and convulsed; eyes shut; he shuts his jaws when he is desired to drink, and appears to feel a little when the left arm is pinched very hard: slight heat of skin; pulse 112, full and regular, (Venæsect, ad. 12 ounces purgative enema, sinapisms, &c.) In the course of the day the patient died in the greatest agony.

" *Autops. cadav.,* — twenty-four hours after death. The arachnoid is adhering in eight or ten places in the superior surface of the brain; in removing it the cortical substance comes away with it in pieces of about the size of a franc, and about a line in thickness; the medullary substance is a little injected. The left lung is a little hard posteriorly, deprived of air, and somewhat hepatized. The right is red, and congested in about the same place. The mucous membrane of the stomach is red in its splenic portion. All the other organs are healthy."

CASE V. — "Antoine Broussart, 65 years of age, having experienced great losses in commerce, and being reduced to great misery, gave himself, on the 6th of January, in the morning, many blows on the head with a

hammer; but not succeeding in killing himself, he takes
a bad pair of scissors, seizes the right testicle with the
left hand, and removes it with the scissors.   This furious
fellow is mastered and is taken to the hospital La Charite.   On the road he tried, but in vain, to strangle himself.   On his arrival the surgeon who was present observed about the line of union of the parietal bones with the
frontal, a considerable tumour, which he opened by a
crucial incision, to allow the extravasated blood to escape,
and to ascertain whether there was any fracture.   The
next day, the 7th, M. Roux examined the wound, and
stated that there was no fracture, and had it dressed in
the ordinary way, as well as that of the scrotum.   (*Low
diet, petit lait emetise.*)   The 8th, no accident has occurred.   The following days the patient was getting better,
when the wound of the head, which till then had secre-
ted a large quantity of pus, began to get dry.   The 20th
he fell into a state of coma; his pulse became hard and
quick, his skin exceedingly hot ; an ichorous matter flowed
from the nostrils.   To this, furious delirium supervenes ;
the patient jumps out of bed, threatens his neighbours,
wishes to fight them, when he is seized by two nurses,
who replace him in bed and tie him to it.   He expires
in a quarter of an hour.

" *Autops. cadav.* — The dura mater, which is thickened, is covered by a yellow false membrane, and on its
internal surface are a few black tubercles ; the pia mater
is equally thickened ; the arachnoid is nearly altogether
disorganized, especially between the convolutions of the
cerebrum, which are bathed with pus ; the superficial
layers of this part are softened and in a state of suppuration: there is nothing else worthy of remark.

" This case confirms what we have already said, viz.
that a circumscribed lesion of the grey substance has no
direct influence on the movements of the extremities."

Other writers incidentally alluding to the diseases of the brain have advanced opinions that confirm the views of M. Foville. Sir Everard Home in his Croonian Lecture, read to the Royal Society, Dec. 7th, 1820, says, " That the cortical part of the brain is the seat of memory, is an opinion I have long entertained, from finding that any continued undue pressure upon the upper anterior part of the brain entirely destroys memory, and a less degree materially diminishes it. Pressure upon the dura mater, where the skull has been trepanned, puts a temporary stop to all sense, which is restored the moment that pressure is removed, and the organ appears to receive no injury from repeated experiments of this kind having been made. In hydrocephalus, when the fluid is in large quantities, and there only remains the cortical part of the brain, and the pons varolii connecting it to the cerebellum, all the functions go on, and the memory can retain passages of poetry, so as to say them by heart; but a violent shake of the head produces instant insensibility. Pressure in a slight degree upon the sinciput, produced in one case complete derangement, with violent excesses of the passion of lust, both of which went off upon removing, by the crown of the trepan, the depressed bone."

Larrey* has also furnished cases of injury of the anterior and superior portions of the brain, producing some intellectual derangement but not affecting motion, and other cases of wounds confined to the base of the brain producing different paralytic affections, but no mental aberrations.

The opinion of M. Foville respecting the functions of the medullary portion of the brain, that it is connected

---

* Clinique Chirurgicale, &c. Par Le Baron Larrey.

with the motive powers and not with the intellectual, is also supported by pathological facts.

CASE VI.—The following case seems to fully establish this opinion, and it is on other accounts one of the most instructive on record ; I do not know of any one more so. It was that of an Idiot, who died during the clinical course of M. Esquirol, in 1823. The right side of the body was exceedingly atrophied. The limbs of this side were reduced almost to skin and bone, and not capable of the least motion. They were also considerably shorter than the limbs of the opposite side, which were well developed and capable of motion. In short the left side of the body was in a natural and healthy condition, while the right was paralytic, emaciated and of diminutive length.

The cause of this singular appearance was sought for after death with great diligence and the autopsy was witnessed by a large number.

No disease was found on examining the body, except that of the brain. The head was quite small, though the bones of the cranium exhibited nothing remarkable. The hemispheres of the brain presented no appearance of convolutions. The cineritious substance was wanting on both sides. But the condition of the medullary part of the brain was most interesting. On the right side it was natural, as the disease appeared to have extended only to the surface of the right hemisphere ; but in the left hemisphere it was almost entirely wanting, and its place filled by a semi-transparent fluid. It is evident from this condition of the brain, that the paralysis and atrophy of the right side of the body was owing to the absence of the medullary portion of the left side of the brain, and that motion cannot be dependent on the cineritious portion of the convolutions for this was wanting on both sides. The absence of the cineritious substance may however account for the idiocy.*

As I have said, I do not know of a case deserving of more consideration than this, not merely as relates to the confirmation of the views advanced respecting the functions of the cineritious and medullary parts of the brain, but as showing that the healthy and full developement of the muscles, limbs, and other parts of the body, is dependent upon the healthy condition of the nervous system; a fact to which I shall again refer.

The conclusions drawn by M. Foville from his observations are, 1st. Morbid alterations of the cineritious portion of the brain are directly connected with derangement of the intellect. 2d. Morbid alterations in the medullary portion are connected with disorder in the motive powers.

My own observations, have convinced me of the general correctness of these observations. I have repeatedly examined the brains of those who died after long continued insanity. In every such case I have witnessed some disease of the cineritious portion of the hemispheres,† sometimes slight and apparently as if produced by extension from the diseased membranes which adhered to the brain. In some cases the medullary portion was harder than natural, but the most marked appearances of disease were in the convolutions of the cerebral lobes, and in none was any disorder of motion manifested. I have also seen extensive disease of the brain, producing convulsions and coma, without mental derangement. The fol- is a case of this kind.

---

* Dic. Med. and Chir. Prat. Vol. 1.

† " Some writers," says Dr. Armstrong, " say they could find no marks of disease in the heads of those who died insane. I must believe their examinations were not critical." I concur in this opinion.

CASE VII. — Mr. C., of Berkshire Co., Mass., aged 30, in the winter of 1818, was supposed to have fallen from a scaffold in his barn, as he was found on the floor in nearly an insensible state. He was however soon aroused, and by the aid of his wife walked to his house. I saw him the same day, no visible injury of the head, complained of pain in the forehead, and was drowsy, but rational, and not in the least paralytic. He was bled and took cathartic medicines, and the next day appeared a little better, but complained of feeling bad. He was able to walk about his room, but with staggering steps as if intoxicated. His countenance had a very anxious appearance, though his intellect was not disturbed. The following night he had a violent convulsive attack, resembling a severe epileptic fit, and was again bled. He now began to be paralytic and comatose, had convulsions every two or three hours, until his death, which occurred on the fifth day.

Dissection. — No appearance of injury externally. On examining the brain no other injury was found than a fracture across the base of the cranium from one ear to the other, and above it three or four ounces of blood extravasated.

Cases similar, or of extensive disease of the base of the brain without producing derangement of the intellect, but causing paralysis and convulsions, are to be found in medical works, some of which will be referred to when treating of the cerebral nerves.

The opinions advanced on this subject are also supported by anatomical facts and argument as follows :—

" A circumstance bearing upon the present question is, that *the grey matter increases in quantity in the exact ratio of the nervous energy.* We learn from a comparative examination of the brain, that the intellectual operations become diversified and energetic in proportion as the grey substance is accumulated ; and that it is in this respect, especially, more than in that of relative volume, that the brains of the lower animals differ when compared with each other, or with the human cerebrum, the great peculiarity of which consists of the very large proportion of its grey matter, when contrasted with the nerves attached to its base. A very accurate test of the intelligence possessed by different animals, and even by different individuals of the human species, is thus afforded by the developement of the convolutions, or, in other words, of the grey substance ; for the so-called convolutions of the brain are only another illustration of that principle, so beautifully displayed in the formation of the glands, according to which the largest possible quantity of materials is contained in the smallest possible space.

But the condition of the cerebro-spinal axis, at the time of birth, affords, perhaps, the most satisfactory evidence on this point. At that period, the grey matter of the cerebrum is well known to be very defective, so much so, indeed, that the convolutions are, as it were, in the first stage of their formation, being only marked out by superficial fissures, almost confined to the surface of the brain ; whilst at this identical period, the spinal cord, owing to the imperfect developement of its fibrous part, (which, as will be subsequently shown, is allied with the exercise of sensation and volition,) contains a larger quantity, proportionally, of grey matter than it does in the adult ; in consequence of which, according to the remark of Professor Arnold, that matter, which in the adult is placed so deeply in the interior, approaches much nearer the external surface. Now at this particular time, the true cerebral functions, consisting of the intellectual faculties, sensation and volition, are almost entirely, if not for a brief period totally wanting ; whilst the true spinal functions are in full activity. It is impossible to adduce any more striking

6*

proof than this, to demonstrate that the extent of the power inherent in the nervous system, depends on the quantity of the grey matter.

Professor Tiedemann, in his valuable work on the developement of the brain, has incidentally mentioned a fact which bears on this inquiry ; he has found that in the torpedo, there is a mass of grey substance placed in connection with the fifth and eighth nerves supplying the electrical organs, larger in size than the cerebellum itself, whilst in the common skaite no such mass exists. An exactly analogous fact is furnished by the comparative anatomy of the lobe of the olfactory nerve ; for, in animals distinguished by the acuteness of their smell, that body is remarkably large when contrasted with those in which that sense is less perfect. The object of such formation cannot be mistaken ; it is evidently to generate power.

Lastly, it may be mentioned in corroboration of the opinion here advanced, that the grey matter is only met with in those parts of the nervous system which are known to be the seat of power ; that is to say, in the encephalon, the spinal cord, and the ganglions ; it is wanting, notwithstanding the assertions of Munro to the contrary, in those parts — namely, the nerves — which are proved not to have the capability of originating power."*

Secondly. — We also learn from pathology that the cerebellum is not connected with the operations of the intellect, but is with voluntary motion ; and probably is essential to its proper and regular manifestations. It also appears to be connected with the sensual propen-

---

* Observations on the Structure and Functions of the Spinal Cord. By R. D. Grainger. London, 1837.

sities, and I have observed that its sympathy with the stomach is greater than between the cerebrum and the stomach, though this may arise from its connection with the Par vagum. Cases are to be found in the writings of Morgagni, Lallemand, Abercrombie, Andral, and in the medical periodicals of late years, of disease of the cerebellum, without any disturbance of mind, but in nearly all of them some disorder of motion occurred; though it is true that in most of these cases the disease did not affect both lobes.

In speaking of the cases of softening of the cerebellum which had come to his knowledge, Andral observes, " Whilst the changes of intelligence were variable, incon- stant, and of little importance, the lesions of motion on the contrary were observed in all the cases except one, and in this it is not quite certain that motion was not interfered with.*

The following case quoted by Abercrombie, confirms the above view.

CASE VIII. — " A woman of 35 ; fixed pain in the back of the head ; walk tremulous and unsteady, like a person balancing a burden on the head ; much throbbing in the head ; hysterical symptoms. Remarkable remis- sion of all the symptoms after the formation of an abscess in the axillia ; but the pain returned when it healed, and increased to tremendous severity, and with remarkable remissions. From two o'clock in the morning till two in the afternoon she was in the greatest agony, lying with her eyes closed, the eyebrows contracted, the hands clenched, and the head immoveable in one position, unable to bear the least noise, or to move a muscle. After two P. M. the symptoms gradually remitted ;

---

* Clinique Medicale.

she took food, and about nine fell asleep, and slept till two, when the paroxysm recurred. As the disease advanced the interval became shorter, and for a fortnight before her death the pain was constant ; senses entire to the last ; palsy of the left leg for three days before death ; duration of the case fourteen months.

Morbid appearances. — A tumor at the base of the cerebellum, growing from both lobes of it, and descending within the dura mater into the spinal canal, as low as the sixth spinal nerve. It was soft like the fœtal brain, and seemed to grow out of the interior of the cerebellum. As it lay along the spinal cord, it rested upon the origin of the nerves, but did not involve them in its substance."*

But the following is one of the most extraordinary cases illustrative of the functions of the cerebellum on record. It was first published by Dr. Combette in the Revue Medicale, and has been quoted by Andral in his lectures.

CASE IX. — *"Complete absence of the Cerebellum, together with the Posterior Peduncles, and protuberances of the Cerebrum, in a young girl who died in her eleventh year.* — Communicated by M. COMBETTE, resident in the hospital of St. Anthony, (Service de M. Kapeler.) — Alexandrine Labrosse was born at Versailles, in May, 1820. Her father possessed a strong and robust constitution, but her mother was weak and unhealthy, and moreover, accustomed to excesses of every description. This child was very feeble when born, but well formed ; she continued extremly delicate and puny, and grew but slowly. She had not cut her first teeth at two years of age, and it was only after she had reached her third year, that she began to lisp a few words. M. Miquel, to whom I am indebted for these particulars, saw her for

* Dr. Latham, Med. and Phys. Jour. July, 1826.

the first time in 1827, when he was informed by her father that she was five years old before she could stand alone. He was astonished at her small size, and remarked particularly the great feebleness of the extremities. This symptom, joined to the want of intelligence in the child, and the impossibility of her articulating a word clearly, had induced M. Miquel to suspect some injury in the brain. He was several times called upon to prescribe for gastro-intestinal irritations, although these presented no remarkable peculiarities. The last time he saw her, which was after her ninth year, he found the pupils extremely dilated, from which he was led to suspect the presence of worms in the intestinal canal. He was about to direct anthelmintics, when the nurse informed him that the little patient kept her hands constantly applied over the genital parts.

" On the 12th of January, 1830, she was admitted into the Hospital des Orphelins, as a forsaken child. Her certificate of admission represented her as paralysed in the abdominal extremities, speaking with difficulty, and that her disease was owing to a fright experienced by her nurse.

" In the letter addressed to the superintendent, requesting her admission, M. Miquel observes, " this little girl, although nine and a half years old, in consequence of the poor nourishment and little care she had received, is scarcely as large as a child of six years : this cause has arrested the developement of both her physical and moral faculties."

" At the time of her entrance into the Orphelins, she was feeble, cachectic, and possessed of very little intelligence. Apparently indifferent to every thing surrounding her, she nevertheless manifested friendship and gratitude for those who rendered her any attentions. When spoken to, she replied with difficulty and hesitation.

Her limbs though extremely feeble, yet allowed her to walk, but she often fell down. She possessed the use of all her senses, eat moderately, and all the functions of nutrition were well performed.

" In the month of January, 1831, when seen by M. Combette, her condition was as follows : Her features indicated a deteriorated constitution, and possessed an air of stupidity. She lay constantly upon her back, with her head inclined to the left side, and she could scarcely move her limbs ; which, however, exhibited no dimuni- tion of sensibility. She had the free use of her hands. Her condition always manifested depression and dulness, and she seemed alike indifferent to both pleasure and pain. When questioned, she replied simply, *yes* or *no*, always however correctly.

" For a long time she had been subject to glandular engorgements about the neck, and especially near the parotids, and for a fortnight had a carbuncle of no great size or violence situated on the right buttock. On the three outermost toes on the same side, there existed an ulceration accompanied by a livid redness, from which there was a very abundant discharge of extremely fœtid pus.

" Towards the middle of February, along with her other infirmities, Alexandrine Labrosse had stomatitis, (as had many other children in the hospital,) complicated with symptoms of enteritis. After this she grew daily more and more feeble, exhausted by an incessant diarrhœa.

" She died on the 25th of March, 1831. Since her death, I have been positively informed, that she was addicted to the habit of masturbation. The sisters have also assured me, that she was subject to epileptic convul- sions, and that a few moments before death, she had experienced a violent general convulsion.

"*Autopsy* thirty hours after death.

"*External Habit.* — Body lank and emaciated. Skin discolored. Large slough over the sacrum. A small livid wound on the right buttock, occasioned by the incisions I had made. The three diseased toes had a blackish and gangrenous appearance. Scrofulous engorgements upon the neck.

"*Head.* — Under the integuments of the cranium near the parietal protuberance of the right side, an ecchymosis existed about the size of a dollar. The cranium was rather thicker than usual. The meninges of the brain appeared healthy. The cerebrum appeared in a natural condition, except that it seemed to me comparatively very large. Dissected subsequently by M. Magendie, a small sanguineous effusion was found in the left posterior lobe, which did not appear to have existed long, and which was not more than two or three lines in diameter. The covering of the cerebellum being divided, the medulla oblongata cut at the occipital foramen, and the encephalic mass raised and inverted — the following appearances were observed :

" A large quantity of serum was discharged, filling the occipital fossæ. In place of the cerebellum, I found a gelatinous membrane of a semicircular form, attached to the medulla oblongata by two membranous and gelatinous peduncles. The one of these on the right side had been torn. Near these peduncles I found two small white isolated masses about the size of a pea. On one of these was found one of the branches of the fourth pair of nerves. The tuberculi quadrigemini were entire. On the posterior and inferior side there was the appearance of erosion, in the midst of which the orifice of the canal of Sylvius appeared. It extended a little upon the medulla oblongata, making a slight alteration in the restiform and in the olivary bodies. The fourth ventricle did not exist. There was no trace of a pons varolii, but without any appearance of want of substance. The anterior pyramidalia terminated in a fork by the cerebral peduncles.

" Of the cerebral nerves, I could only find the origin of the first, second, third and fourth pair, which appeared in healthy state, except the latter, which was, as I have said, detached with the small white mass, of which I have spoken. Not having raised the brain myself, it was impossible for me to find the origin of the other pairs. They all, however, existed, and could be easily perceived through the openings of the dura mater. They, have moreover, been subsequently dissected by M. Magendie, and exhibited no peculiarity.

" The cerebral substance was of the ordinary consistence, but the medulla oblongata appeared a little softened, especially about the erosion I have described, where there existed a kind of maceration. The occipital hollows were regularly formed, but appeared to me rather smaller than natural. The vertebral arteries existed. I cannot say how these were distributed, because they did not at first fix my attention.

" *Spine.* — A considerable quantity of serum ran from the spinal canal. The spinal marrow offered nothing remarkable.

" *Chest.* — Both lobes of the lungs crepitated, but their whole surface was covered with miliary tubercles, which were also found in the parenchyma. The cavity of each pleura contained two or three ounces of serosity. The pericardium and heart offered nothing in particular.

" *Abdomen.* — The intestinal circumvolutions were of a deep red color. The mucous membrane of the stomach exhibited a number of red dots on a slate-colored ground, and near the anterior part and great arch, there were five or six brown patches. In the middle of each of these, a small ulceration with elevated and perpendicular borders appeared. This membrane was otherwise of its ordinary consistence and thickness.

" The mucous coat of the duodenum presented no ulceration. It was slightly red, and its follicles prominent. After this, throughout the whole tract of the small intestine, it was of a livid red color, presenting numerous ulcerations, especially about the ileo-cœcal valve. The large intestines presented nothing in particular.

" The mesenteric ganglions were larger than ordinary. The liver was of an extraordinary size, and of a pale color.

"*The Organs of Generation.* — The finger could readily be introduced into the vagina. The hymen did not exist. The labia were of a lively red color, and bore the appearance of having been frequently irritated. The ovaries and uterus existed, but they appeared smaller than usual with girls of the same age.

" The kidneys, spleen, &c. were in a natural state.

" *Conclusions.* — This singular case is calculated to excite the particular attention of physicians of the physiological school, and presents no less interest for pathologists. I regret exceedingly, my inability to say anything relative to the moral condition of this child previous to its entrance into the hospital, and am still in the expectation of receiving further information. Should any particulars be offered, I shall immediately communicate them."*

That the cerebellum is not concerned in intellectual operations is evident from the fact that inflammation of the arachnoid membrane over it, does not produce delirium, while it is well known that inflammation of this

---

* Bull. de la Soc. Anat. — Rev. Medicale, April, 1831.

membrane covering the cerebral hemispheres produces violent raving. Such instances have been given by Recamier, Martinet and others.* The following from Abercrombie is to a like purpose.

Case X. — " A lady, 45, liable to suppuration of the left ear, complained of pain in that ear, May 11, 1821. On the two following days, the pain extended through the head with fever ; and on the 14th, she complained of general headache, and a violent and painful feeling of throbbing in the back part of the head. She was deaf, and inclined to drowsiness, but quite sensible ; pulse 120 and very strong ; large blood-letting and the other usual remedies were actively employed on this and the following days by Dr. Thatcher and the late Mr. Bryce. I saw her on the 16th ; there was then a good deal of coma, but she was sensible when roused ; the eye natural, the tongue clean, pulse 130 ; she still complained of headache when she was closely questioned, but did not make any complaint except when she was much roused. The pulse being now considerably reduced in strength, topical bleeding only was employed. In the evening she was more easily roused, and said she felt better ; in the night she became again extremely restless and incoherent, and died early in the morning. There had been a slight discharge of matter from the left ear early in the disease.

" *Inspection.* — There was slight effusion in the lateral ventricles ; the brain in other respects was healthy. On the outer surface of the cerebellum there was a uniform deposition of thick puriform matter ; it was most abundant on the left side. The pia mater of the cerebellum was highly vascular, the dura mater was healthy : there

---

* Revue Medicale, 1823.

was some purulent matter about the pituitary gland, and in the cavity of the ear, but there was no appearance of disease of the bones connected with the ear, or of the dura mater covering them."

That some part of the cerebellum is connected with the motive powers, is rendered probable from the fact, that in nearly all the cases on record of disease of this part of the brain, some disorder of motion was observed. This is the most common symptom in disease of this organ. Still the effect of disease of the cerebellum upon the motive powers varies very much. Generally there is a paralysis of the opposite side, sometimes a staggering like drunkenness, and sometimes only strabismus is noticed, and in some instances no disorder of motion at all, as the following cases show.

CASE XI. — *An abscess in the cerebellum and rupture of the lateral sinus by Mr. John Douglass, Surgeon in Edinburgh.* G. B. aged 19 years, was taken with a pain and heaviness in the forehead, for which he was plentifully blooded, vomited, purged, blistered, &c.. Notwithstanding which he was obliged to sit always with his head leaning forward, otherwise his pain was greatly increased. His pulse in the mean time was good, he had no convulsions, but his appetite was bad, his sleep broken, and in turning his eyes quickly, he had an addition of pain.

After being three months in this way, he became free from pain, in an evening in the beginning of January 1737, eat the wing of a hen, drank a glass of strong ale, after which he slept well all night, next morning he called for tea, and immediately after fell into a seeming faint, just as I happened to enter his lodging. 1 opened a vein in his arm, but he did not bleed, and in two minutes he died.

When his head was opened, we saw two ounces of

perfect pus contained in a suppurated tumor formed in the middle of the cerebellum, and an opening of the left lateral sinus of the dura mater, out of which a considerable quantity of blood had flowed.*

In this case it will be observed, no mention is made of paralysis or disturbance of the motive powers.

In the 22d vol. of the Lancet, is a case quoted from the clinical lectures of the Baron Dupuytren, of a serous cyst developed in the right lobe of the cerebellum which lobe had entirely disappeared, without any alteration in the cerebral or general functions.   In the 17th volume of the Lancet is the following case.

CASE XII. — *Abscess in the cerebellum.*   Eliza Purt, aged 19, was admitted into Faith's Ward, St. Bartholomew's Hospital, on the 13th of January, under the care of Mr. Lawrence.   She has paralysis of the portio dura of the right side ; during sleep the eyelid of the affected side is but half closed ; and when she laughs, the muscles of that side remain motionless, and thus a rather ludicrous appearance is produced.   She suffers severe pain in her head, but none of the functions of the body are disturbed.   There are two excrescences in the meatus auditorius externus of the right side, attended with purulent discharge.   She states that she has been subject to headache for the last twelve months, and that lately excressences have appeared in the meatus.   She has been married a fortnight, since which the pain in her head has increased to such an extent, as to compel her to come here to seek relief.

The treatment which was adopted was antiphlogistic, and consisted of five copious bleedings from the arm, the

---

* Edinburgh Medical Essays, Vol. V. Part II.

application of leeches to the head, a blister to the nape of the neck, and active purging. These remedies were attended with considerable mitigations of her sufferings ; a portion of one of the excrescences came away, which also was productive of relief. The pain being still severe her head was shaved, and ice applied to it. She was then submitted to a course of mercury, which affected her system in a few days. These measures were not capable of arresting the disease, and she died on the 27th of January.

Post-Mortem Examination, seven hours after death.

Head. — Membranes of the brain perfectly healthy, the convolutions appeared paler than usual, and were much flattened, especially on the right side. There were no evidences of inflammation in the substance of the brain. Three ounces of very transparent fluid were found in the lateral ventricles. On dividing the tentorium, the right half of the cerebellum appeared enlarged, and its anterior part felt as if it contained fluid. When it was cut into, about half an ounce of thin, and very fetid pus escaped ; the parietes of the abscess were of a blackish-green color, and the cerebellum was adherent to the meatus auditorius internus. On stripping off the dura mater from the petrous portion of the temporal bone, thick pus was seen on the upper surface of the superior wall of the tympanum. This was washed off, and ulceration of the bone beneath it was observed ; there was an opening in it, through which a probe was passed into the tympanum, which when its superior wall was removed, was found full of pus. There were two excrescences in the meatus auditorius externus ; one attached to the lower part of the meatus, the other to the membrani tympani, and in this membrane were several small holes. The portio dura was examined and exhibited its

7*

usual appearance. The thoracic and abdominal viscera were healthy. The uterus and ovaries were enlarged and in a state of congestion, and in the right ovary a very beautiful corpus luteum was found.

In the third volume of the American Journal of the Medical Sciences is an interesting account of disease of the cerebellum by John Ware, M. D. of Boston. It is briefly as follows.

CASE XIII. — A lad ten years of age complained for some months of very severe pains in the head, recurring in paroxysms, and produced by the least irregularity or improper indulgence in eating. The stomach was extremely irritable and vomiting often occurred. For a short time he appeared to amend, but owing apparently to eating of some indigestible food his paroxysms of pain returned, and he was finally seized of convulsions, and died in eighteen hours.

Appearances on Dissection. The veins of the pia mater were unusually vascular, and five or six ounces of a straw colored fluid was found in the lateral ventricles.

" The fornix, septum lucidum, and the thalami were unusually firm, and of unusual whiteness. The consistence of the other parts of the cerebrum was natural ; numerous red points presented wherever an incision was made. On dividing the tentorium slight adhesions were found between this and the cerebellum. On the left crus cerebelli between the arachnoid and pia mater, a small globular tumor, was seen, one third of an inch in diameter, of the consistence of the cortical substance, and of a granulated texture. On the inferior surface of the tentorium, near its attachment to the petrous portion of the temporal bone, on the left side, was a bilobated tumor, very firmly adherent, of firm consistence, of an oval form, about one inch in length. In the left lobe of the cerebellum there were two, and in the right lobe three round tumors from one-half to three-fourths of an inch in diameter. On dividing one of them it was found to consist of a firm cyst, containing a substance of a greenish-yellow color, similar in its external characters to the matter found in encysted tubercles of the lungs. These tumors were imbedded in the convolutions of the cerebellum, and by care could be removed without destroying the texture of the parts. Those in the left lobe were less firmly attached to the pia mater than those in the right. The substance of the cerebellum appeared less firm than natural, but no *ramollisement* existed around the tumours. The pia mater of the medulla oblongata was considerably injected, and a small quantity of serous fluid was found at the base of the brain. The thorax and abdomen were not examined.

"During the whole course of this disease says Dr. W., the functions of the brain were unaffected in a remarkable degree. There was no failure of the powers of the intellect, memory, sensation, speech, or motion. There was never any thing peculiar in his gait; his manner of walking at different times was determined wholly by the amount of his muscular strength. He moved precisely as any other person would do who was equally weak. His countenance was melancholly and his eye rather heavy. He was generally silent and depressed, and easily moved to tears by very slight causes."

By some the cerebellum has been considered the organ of the sensual propensities. Dr. Gall was the first I believe who advanced this opinion, though he does not consider, as I have already shown by a quotation from his writings, that the cerebellum has no other function.

That some part of the cerebellum is appropriated to, or is the seat of this propensity, I believe we must admit, as the cases are very numerous of disease of this organ

affecting the genital organs. I will refer to some of
them.

The following is from Hennen's Principles of Military
Surgery.

CASE XIV. — Gaetano, a soldier of the ninth Portuguese Cacadores, was struck by a piece of shell at
Salamanca, in June, 1813. It shattered the superior part
of the occipital bone from within half an inch of the
great knob on the left side, to the lambdoidal suture.
An irregular angular portion of the left parietal bone,
nearly an inch in length and about an inch in breadth,
was also fractured and beaten inwards. He labored
under most alarming symptoms, total insensibility, involuntary discharge of feces, laborious breathing, irritabilty
of pupil, and weak low pulse with occasional convulsive
twitchings. The removal of the depressed portions of
bone, and about an ounce of coagulum from the surface
of the dura mater, on the second day after the wound,
was attended with a diminution of most of the symptoms ;
and with two copious bleedings, (which were employed to
arrest approaching inflammation,) his recovery was per-
fected by the November following ; except that even then,
the catheter was occasionally necessary to draw off his
urine, the bladder not having recovered from a paralysis,
which, for the first three weeks, was so complete as to
prevent any evacuation without the use of an instrument.
Of this, however he ultimately recovered. This man
was subsequently attached to the mule with my medical
stores, and repeatedly consulted me on the means of
recovering his virility, which, he said, the shell had *completely carried away with it.*

Dr. Hennen adds, " Loss of the generative faculty and
atrophy of the organs connected with it have been
attributed to blows on the back of the head. The fact

is certain, but whether this proceeds from injury to the organs of sensual love, or to a general loss of power, is a subject for future inquiry."

"Priapism is occasionally observed to occur in wounds of the head. In a case which lately occurred in the cavalry hospital near Edinburg, this symptom was particularly remarked in a hussar, who had suffered severe injury by a fall from his horse. The penis was in a state of priapism during the greater part of the two first days after the accident and towards the close of life he frequently rubbed the genitals violently with his hand. On dissection the dura mater was found extensively separated over the head. This separation included the *tentorium cerebelli*, and beneath its edge about four drachms of coagulated blood were found, the principal part of which lay on the cerebellum."

Baron Larrey has furnished several cases showing that the cerebellum and the testicles act and react on each other in disease. "The genital organs seem to have a marked influence upon the cerebellum, for when they are removed by disease, or any other means, the occipital region of the cranium, and cerebellum gradually experience such a sensible reduction, that the occipital bumps which had been more or less protuberant before, disappear, and the whole occipital region of the head is diminished in proportion. We have verified this change of dimension in a great number of soldiers, who had been operated upon for sarcocele, and when one testicle only was removed, there was only a reduction of that portion of the cerebellum and occipital bump, which belonged to the same side with the extirpated testicle."* He mentions this case.

---

* Clinique Chirurgicale, &c. Par Le Baron Larrey.

Case XV. — A soldier, who had been wounded in the occipital region by a splinter of wood, was attacked by all the symptoms of inflamed cerebellum, and in despite of every thing that was done, they were only dissipated by the appearance of an abscess in the nape, which opened spontaneously. In about three months after the accident he rejoined his regiment, and many years elapsed before he again came under Larrey's notice. He was then so extremely altered in appearance, that the author mistook him for a young conscript, who had been exhausted by some asthenic disease. He was thirty-two years of age, of middle size, but thin and pale, his eyes were depressed, his lips blanched, his hair, more especially that which covered his occiput was thin and bristled, and a feeling of pain and coldness was always experienced in the back part of his head. He was beardless, his voice was feminine, and some of the assistants were not without suspicion of his sex, a more minute examination was considered necessary. " To our great surprise," says Larrey, " we found his genital organs reduced to the size of those of an infant some months old. His penis was not more than five or six lines long, and two or three lines thick, it never exhibited any degree of erection, and his testicles were so wasted as scarcely to equal in size a small bean."

Other cases are given by him which I think fully establish an intimate connection between the cerebellum and the genital organs.

Dr. Rowel observed, at the hospital St. Antoine, an apoplectic female, seventy years of age. He remarked that menstruation which had ceased many years before, re-appeared during the course of the disease. From this circumstrnce he concluded that the apoplexy might be cerebellal ; this was found to be the fact, and the uterus was filled with coagulated blood, and its tissue, as well as that of the fallopian tubes and ovaries, was phlogosed.

" A girl, abandoned to a premature indulgence in venereal pleasures, prostrated herself to satisfy her desires, *et se livre a toutes les manœuvres de la masturbation.* She fell into a state of nymphomania. She died, and an induration of the middle lobe of the cerebellum was found, with other appearances of chronic inflammation of the part."*

It is a curious but well-established fact, that hanging produces very frequently, if not usually, priapism and emission. Some infatuated beings have had recourse to suspension by the neck to produce those pleasures they have been unable to obtain by natural means. M. de Seze gives instances of this. The following was related to Mr. Levison by Dr. Travis of Scarborough.

CASE XVI. — " Some few years past an Italian *Castrata* singer at the opera was found suspended by the bedstead, and when a surgeon was called in *the man was dead*, although (as stated by the landlady of the house,) he had hung himself unintentionally. The facts of the transaction were thus stated by this woman to he jury summoned to sit on the body ; she said ' that the deceased had informed her, (when he came to lodge at her house) that he had been deprived, in the most barbarous manner, of certain essential parts for sexual gratification, but that *at certain times* he experienced a very powerful desire, and that he had accidentally discovered that by partially hanging himself he allayed the desire, and had certain delightful sensations,' and she assured the jury that she had been in the habit of cutting him down on many occasions ; and that during his last

* Lancet, Vol. 19.

pleasurable suspension she had heard a rapping at her street door, and ran down to answer it, but although she returned as quickly as possible, the gentleman's life was gone, &c. The medical gentleman called on the same occasion informed the jury, that as all executed criminals had priapism and emission, the account given of the *Castrata* was not improbable."*

On the connection which exists between the cerebellum and the genital organs, Dr. Carswell, after stating that many cases have been recorded which prove that a functional relation exists between the cerebellum and testes, says, that he has " met with two cases in particular, in which this relationship was manifested in a most remarkable manner. They occurred in two young men, from eighteen to twenty years of age, who reduced themselves to a state of the most appalling moral and physical degradation by the act of self-pollution. Both of them died from its effects ; one of them having often declared that he was compelled towards the gratification of a desire which he had no power to control, for he had frequently attempted the consummation of it after the prepuce had been excised as a means of prevention, and when the glans and part of the penis were in a state of active inflammation. In each of these patients the cerebellum was the seat of a tumor as large as a hen's egg, composed entirely of the medullary sarcoma."†

In Meckel's Archives of Physiology, for 1823, are detailed the particulars of the case of a boy two years of age, in whom a premature developement of the genital organs and of the occipital region was contemporaneous. M. Serres has related some cases of chronic

---

* Lancet, Vol. 19, p. 49.

† Illustrations of the Elementary Forms of Disease. By Robert Carswell, M. D.

inflammation and congestion of the cerebellum, in which erection of the penis was a constant symptom. Andral refers to cases of diseased cerebellum, accompanied by partial erection of the penis and erotic delirium. M. Menard enumerates priapism among the symptoms characteristic of inflammation of the cerebellum.

In support of this view of the seat of the sexual propensity, are cases of recovery from Nymphomania and Masturbation by remedies applied to the occipital region. Levison refers to a case of Nymphomania, cured by shaving the back of the head and applying ice over the cerebellar region. The cure was rapid and complete. In the Gazette Medicale of Paris, 1835, M. St. Martin, writes from Turin, that Ferroresi cured a young girl afflicted with violent Nymphomania, and two young men who suffered from the incorrigible habit of masturbation by the application of ice to the back of the head over the region of the cerebellum.

The cerebellum of a young man long addicted to the habit of masturbation, was found, by Dr. Fuller, Physician to the Retreat for the Insane, in this city, diminished and diseased.

It appears also from pathological researches, that a close sympathy exists between the cerebellum and the stomach. In a former publication, I endeavored to show that many cases of indigestion or dyspepsia as the complaint is termed, arise from functional or organic disease of the brain. Every year's experience confirms me in the correctness of this opinion. But it appears to me that disease of the cerebellum more frequently affects the stomach, than disease of the cerebrum. Is it in consequence of the diseases of the cerebellum affecting the origin of the Par Vagum?

Cases like the following are not unfrequently seen.

8

CASE XVII. — " A medical man in the meridian of life, had been for a year liable to attacks of dyspepsia, with headache. In October, 1815, he had severe headach with fever, relieved by blood-letting : then complete want of digestion, headache, general emaciation, and frequent vomiting, which occurred chiefly in the morning. He had various uneasy feelings, which he referred to his liver, and his complaints were ascribed to this source by the most eminent practitioners whom he consulted. In August 1816, he had severe headache, and nothing agreed with his stomach ; almost every thing being vomited. After some time, the pain was relieved, but the morning sickness and vomiting continued, with increasing emaciation, torpid bowels, frequent eructations, and hiccup. In the end of September, had twice a slight convulsion. Headache then periodical — mind entire, but conversation induced headache, and sometimes convulsion. October 9, died suddenly in convulsion.

Morbid Appearances. — " Four ounces of fluid in the ventricles. On the inferior part of the left lobe of the cerebellum, there was an encysted tumor, the size of a French walnut, besides a vesicular portion connected with it containing some yellow serum. The tumor was invested both by the dura mater, and pia mater, and was attached by a small pedicle to the substance of the cerebellum, where it had formed a depression in which it was embedded. On the corresponding part of the opposite lobe, there was a small florid tumor the size of a large pea. The abdominal viscera were sound."*

From these pathological facts, it is evident that we have not as yet fully ascertained the functions of the cerebellum. It is not to my mind, quite apparent that the cases quoted of disease of the cerebellum producing paralysis,

---

* Med. Repos. Vol. VII.

establishes the fact. The paralysis might have arisen from pressure or irritation of the medulla oblongata or the crura cerebri. Besides there has occurred extensive disease of the cerebellum, without disorder of motion. Some such cases have been already quoted, and others might be added. One thing is very remarkable, that when disease occurs in the cerebrum, and in the cerebellum of the opposite side, the paralysis is always opposite to the side of the diseased cerebrum. The affection of the cerebellum appears in such cases to have no influence.

Andral alludes to this fact in his section on " Hemorrhage of the Cerebellum." " When the hemorrhage of the cerebellum occurs simultaneously with that of the cerebrum, or a little time after it, but so that the blood is effused on the right into the cerebellum, and on the left into the cerebrum, or *vice versa*, there is paralysis only on the side of the body opposite to the hemisphere of the cerebrum in which the hemorrhage has taken place, that is, on the same side as the hæmorrhage of the cerebellum, How then does it come to pass that, whereas the movement of the extremities of the right side are abolished in consequence of an effusion of blood in the left hemisphere of the cerebrum, the effusion which takes place simultaneously into the right hemisphere of the cerebellum, has no longer the power of paralysing the extremities of the left side ?"

The following are interesting cases illustrative of the same fact.

CASE XVIII. — *Atrophy of one half of the Encephalon.* This case was communicated to the Anatomical Society of Paris, by M. Bodey, and shows that a single lobe suffices for the integrity of the intellectual faculties. The *left* lobe was atrophied, reduced to half its original volume, composed of close circonvolutions, small and slightly in-

durated, and had lost the faculty of controlling the movements of the right side of the body.   The left side of the
cranium was considerably thickened, and the serosity accumulated in the correspondent lateral ventricle, had filled the void left by the gradual atrophy of the cerebral
substance.   The left peduncle of the brain had suffered
a diminution of volume proportioned to the lessening of
the lobe which it supported, a fact which astonishes no
one at present, but which Bichat had difficulty in recon-
ciling with his refusal to admit the fibrous structure of the
encephalon.   The intelligence in this case remained unaffected.   In this same subject, one of the hemispheres of
the cerebellum, was atrophied, but what is singular is,
that while the *left* lobe of the cerebrum was effected, it
was the *right* hemisphere of the cerebellum, that was
atrophied."*

CASE XIX. — A man 42 years of age, died at the Hotel Dieu, on the 13th of April, two days after his admis,
sion, under symptoms of disease of the heart.   He had
from his infancy been affected with complete hemiplegia of the right side ; the paralysed limbs were atrophic
and the phalanges of the fingers dislocated backwards ;
the intellectual faculties, and the functions of the external
senses were not in the least impaired.

On post mortem examination, the lower extremities,
were found infiltrated ; the pleura and peritoneum contained a considerable quantity of serum, and the left ventricle of the heart was hypertrophied.   The most remarkable alteration was, however, observed in the brain ;
the left half of the skull was twice as thick as the right,
and the left hemisphere of the brain was accordingly
much depressed, the right anterior lobe was larger than

* Review Medicale, 1830.

the left by half an inch ; the convolutions of the left hemisphere were attenuated, flattened, of unusual consistence, and white color ; the left lateral ventricle contained a large quantity of serum ; its parieties were so thin as to resemble a membrane ; the left thalamus opticus, corpus striatum, crus cerebri, and the left portion of the pons varolii, were atrophic. The alteration of the cerebellum was the inverse of that of the brain, its right hemisphere being atrophic, and smaller by a third than the left. This remarkable case having been read at the Academie Royale de Medicine, by M. Gueneau de Mussy, under whose care the patient had been at the Hotel Dieu.

M. Amussat remarked that he had observed several cases of atrophy of one of the hemispheres, and that in all of them the opposite half of the cerebellum had been atrophic.

M. Ferrus made the same remark; in some of his cases, however, the same side of the cerebellum had been atrophic, and most of the patients had been idiots, one of them, however, in whom the left hemisphere was found destroyed, and replaced by a small quantity of pulpeous matter, had up to the period of his death been in the full enjoyment of his senses and mental faculties."*

All that we can properly conclude at the present time respecting the cerebellum and its functions, is, that this organ is not concerned in the operations of the intellect, but some part of it appears to be with the motive powers, and also some portions of it with the sexual propensity.   The close sympathy between the cerebellum and the stomach, is a fact deserving of attention.

Thirdly. — Pathology also teaches us that the integrity of one hemisphere of the brain is alone sufficient for the

---

* Lancet, Vol. xvi. p. 495.

8*

manifestation of the mental powers.   Cases are quite numerous in medical works of extensive disease of one of
the hemispheres, without any mental disturbance.   I have
seen such myself and some have already been quoted.   I
will refer but to a few more, and those the most remarkable.   A man mentioned by Dr. Ferriar,* died of disease of the head, retaining his faculties entire, until the
moment of his death, which was sudden.   On examining the brain the whole of the right hemisphere was
found destroyed by suppuration.   Mr. O'Halloran,† relates the case of a man who from injury of the head had
a large piece of bone removed on the right side, from
which a great quantity of pus mixed with the substance
of the brain was discharged.   Mr. O'Halloran affirms
that three ounces of brain were discharged at a dressing,
and that the cavern in the brain was terrible.   The patient lived to the seventeenth day, and though paralytic
on the left side, retained his intellect until the moment of
his death.   In the fifth volume of the Memoirs of the Med-
cal Society of London, for 1798, is a case furnished by
Mr. Waldron, and communicated to the Society by Mr.
Abernethy, of a gun breech above three inches long, and
weighing three ounces and a drachm, penetrating the
cranium over the right side, above the frontal sinus, and
remaining imbedded in the right hemisphere for two
months, without producing disorder of the intellect.   The
case is certainly very extraordinary, and is detailed at
great length and drawings given of the gun breech in the
work to which I have referred.

The following is from Andral.

CASE XX. — A man, twenty eight years of age, fell

---

* Manchester Memoirs, Vol, iv,

† Injuries of the head.

when three years old, from the first story into the street, on his head. After this fall he remained paralysed on the left side. By degrees an habitual extension of the left foot on the leg was established so that on this side he walked only on the point of the foot. The left upper extremity was completely deprived of motion ; no trace of contraction any where observed. The person had some education, and had profited by it; he had a good memory ; speech perfectly free ; and his intellect such as is ordinarily met with in the generality of persons. Having entered the infirmary of Bicetre, where he lived, for a chronic affection of the chest, he was there seized with symptoms of acute peritonitis, of which he died.

Post Mortem. — The vault of the cranium having been removed, the meninges of the right side were found transparent, and fluctuating through almost their entire extent. They were cut into, and a clear limpid serum like spring water, gushed forth. Between these meninges and the ventricles there existed not the slightest trace of nervous substance. These membranes constituted the upper wall of an immense cavity, the lower side of which was formed by the optic *thalamus,* the *corpus striatum,* and all the other parts situate, on the level of these two bodies. Of the nervous mass above the ventricles there remained only that which, being anterior to the *corpus striatum,* forms its anterior wall. Numerous tubercles were in the two lungs, and several ulcerations appeared on the surface of the small intestine. There was a perforation in the ileum, whence the peritonitis which terminated the life of the patient.

Remarks. — The lesion, discovered in this case, began from external violence, twenty-five years before the period when it came under our inspection. The atrophy of the brain was not probable here the primitive alteration ; it succeeded to other changes of an inflamatory nature which supervened immediately after the fall.

The perfect preservation of the intellect up to the last moment is certainly a remarkable circumstance in a case where so great a portion of the brain had for a long time been removed.

The same fact is proved by the effects of inflammation of one of the hemispheres of the cerebrum.

" When inflammation," says Bouillaud, " only occupies a part, more or less extensive, of one of the cerebral hemispheres, and when the other hemisphere is in a healthy state, the intellectual and moral functions. at least ordinarily, present no notable lesion. It seems that in this case the healthy hemisphere suffices for the exercise of these functions. But if the inflammation of one hemisphere spreads itself over the other hemisphere, a *delirium* of variable form occurs, according to the extent and intensity of the inflammation, and perhaps also according to the part affected either in one or the other hemisphere. A general delirium always exists when the partial irritation generalizes itself, an accident unfortunately often seen."

I might multiply proof to any extent, that when only one hemisphere of the brain is diseased, even to a great degree, the intellectual faculties many remain undisturbed. It is true however, that in many cases when only one hemisphere appears to be effected, derangement or loss of the mental powers is observed. This undoubtedly arises from the extension of inflammation or irritation from the opposite hemisphere.

Not unfrequently when a discharge is kept up from the brain by an opening in the cranium on one side, the intellect is not disturbed, but when the discharge is prevented, coma and loss of intelligence supervene.

It will be noticed that in all these cases, one hemisphere remained unaffected, but I am not aware that there is a single well authenticated case of both hemispheres being much injured without mental disturbance. Solly observes, " there are no cases on record in which the mental faculties have remained undisturbed, where disorganization of the brain extended to both hemispheres." I apprehend the mind is often considered sound when it is not so. If after an injury of the head, the patient knows his former acquaintance and answers correctly a few questions, and does not rave, he is said to have no disturbance of the intellect, but in such instances some of the mental powers may be disordered, notwithstanding it is unnoticed by inattentive observers.

I have seen such. I have often seen persons after severe injury of the head, answer most questions correctly, know their acquaintances readily, and deemed by their friends to have no disturbance of mind, while a closer scrutiny has convinced me that this conclusion was incorrect.

That many of the mental faculties remain undisturbed when considerable disease of the brain exists, is not more surprising than that the power of digestion remains, as we know it often does, when the stomach is much diseased. Neither on the other hand, is it surprising that a very little disease of the brain, a trifle of inflammation of one hemisphere should sometimes disturb the intellect, when we consider the close connexion of all parts of the brain, and its enclosure in a solid case which it completely fills, and consequently cannot be much affected in one part without other parts being disturbed and irritated.

Here I wish to lay down a few principles which ought to guide us in studying the functions of the brain by the aid of pathological researches.

First.—We may not always attribute all the symptoms noticed in a case of injury of the brain, to disturbance of the functions of the particular part of the brain injured ; for the injury itself may disturb the functions of other portions of the brain. Nevertheless, numerous cases of injury or disease of the same parts of the brain, followed by similar mental disturbance, might justify us in concluding that the injured parts were especially devoted to the manifestation of the mental powers now affected.

Second. — When we find certain mental faculties not disturbed by an injury extending to corresponding parts of both hemispheres, we have a right to conclude that the portion of brain injured is not essential to the manifestation of these faculties. For instance, when we find both sides of the cerebellum wholly disorganized, or the pons varolii, medulla oblongata, fornix, pineal gland, &c., without any disturbance of the mind, we may conclude that these parts are not essential to mental action ; and this conclusion is not overthrown by cases of disease of these parts, accompanied by disorder of the intellect, for in the latter cases the disorder of the intellect might arise from functional disorder produced in other portions of the brain from the organic disease of the parts we have mentioned.

Fourthly. — Pathological investigations have not only shown us that different parts of the brain have different functions, but have rendered it probable that the anterior lobes of the brain are the seat of the more important of the intellectual faculties. " M. Breschet," says Andral, " has published the remarkable case of a girl fifteen years of age, in whom the two anterior lobes were wanting. At the bottom of, and behind, the membranous pouch which replaced them, the two *corpus striata* were seen exposed. The head was very well formed.

The girl was plunged into a complete state of idiocy ; it was necessary to dress her and feed her ; she was averse to walk, though she had the power of moving all her limbs with ease, and with equal facility ; she was usually sitting, and remained so for entire days, alternately inclining the head from one shoulder to the other ; vision was entire ; the most perfect indifference existed for the quality of odors."

In the 14th volume of the *Medico Chirurgical Review* is the following notice of a case of *congenital absence of the anterior lobes of the brain.* " In the Annual Report of the new Anatomical Society of Paris, a preparation was shown by M. Lacroix, exemplifying the above mal-organization. The secretary of the society makes use of the following words : ' If the opinion which assigns to the anterior lobes of the brain the privilege of presiding over the higher intellectual operations, needed any new confirmation, it would find a powerful argument in its favor in the case reported by M. Lacroix. In that case there was a complete congenital absence of the anterior lobes of the cerebrum, which were replaced by a collection of transparent serum, communicating freely with the ventricles. This physical condition was accompanied, not by a perversion, but by an almost entire nullity of the intellect and moral functions. Here was an experiment made by nature, more valuable for physiology than any vivisections of the anatomist.' The secretary remarks that this case tells both for and against the phrenologists ; for them, as showing the seat of intelligence to be in the anterior part of the brain ; against them, as showing that their skill could not have detected the cause of the idiocy, since the forehead was well formed, though full of water, and all the prominences well marked.

Almost at the same time that the above preparation was shown, another came under view, where the left hemisphere of the brain was found atrophied to one half its original volume, without any loss of intellectual faculties, the other lobe being entire. The atrophy was occasioned by an accumulation of fluid in the lateral ventricle of the side, and the opposite half of the body was completely paralytic."

Otto remarks in his compendium of Pathological Anatomy that in idiots the front lobes are usually small and shallow. This is confirmed by the observation of others. I do not know of any case on record of the anterior lobes of the brain being diseased without manifest disturbance of the intellect, but cases of disease of portions of both posterior lobes have been witnessed without producing any noticeable change in the mental powers. The following is an instance of the kind, taken from the *Medico Chirurgical Review* for Oct. 1826.

CASE XXI. — Dr. Chambers has reported, in our respected cotemporary, the case of a woman, Mrs. Miles, whom we attended previously to her admission into St. George's Hospital. When she first applied to us, she complained of discharges of blood from the lungs by coughing. This was stopped by a few doses of super-acetate of lead and opium. She next complained of sickness at stomach, whenever she took food, together with pain in the occipital region of the head. Blisters were applied to both parts, and medicines were given to quiet the gastric irritability, but without success. The patient having but bad accommodations in the Little Theatre of the Hay-market, we sent her to St. George's Hospital. There the sickness at stomach and pain of the head were treated with the same want of success as before. There was no tenderness of the epigastrium or abdomen, pulse from 80 to 90, tongue clean, skin cool, bowels constipated. The intellectual functions were never disturbed. Among the remedial agents, she was placed under the full influence of mercury ; an issue was inserted in the back of her head ; blisters were applied to her epigastrium ; opium, subnitrate of bismuth, &c. were given internally, but all to no purpose. At length she died exhausted by the progressive increase of the symptoms. Some curious speculations were hazarded as to the nature of the disease, and one gentleman, who could see deeper than the rest, considered it as a tuberculation of the peritoneum. It was *not* Dr. Chambers.

On dissection, no diseased appearance was found in the stomach or bowels. In the centre of the posterior lobe of the right hemisphere of the brain was a small tumor, the size of a large nut, somewhat softer than the contiguous brain. A similar mass was found in the posterior lobe of the left hemisphere. The left lobe of the cerebellum was almost entirely destroyed by the suppurative softening of a similar tumor occupying its interior. The surrounding cerebellic substance was softened, and there were three ounces of water in the ventricles."

This case illustrates well the sympathetic effects of cerebral disease on the stomach. It was of the latter organ that the patient chiefly complained. With all this organic disease of the brain, the intellect was unimpaired to the last. I apprehend that the grey substance of the cerebrum was not affected, and that the disease of the cerebellum caused the sympathetic disease of the stomach.

Other cases might here be referred to, showing that wounds of the anterior lobes of the brain sometimes produce loss of the memory of words, numbers, colors, events, &c, but these will be adduced in another place.

Has pathology thrown any light upon the functions of other parts of the brain ?

9

M. Foville* says that lesions of the thalamus nervi optici and its radiations are accompanied by loss of motion in the arms, and that lesions of the corpus striatum and its radiations by derangement of motion in the lower extremities. The same opinion has been advanced by M. Bouillaud.†

Andral objects to these conclusions, and refers to cases that show their incorrectness. One thing appears to be certain that these parts of the cerebrum, the corpora Striata, and thalami, are more frequently found diseased, softened and disorganized by hæmorrhage than any other parts of the brain, and in such cases some disorder of the motive powers is the consequence. Sometimes however in such cases the intellect is not disturbed.

From the fact that each limb may be separately convulsed and palsied, it is probable that different parts of the brain preside over the motions of the upper and lower extremities; and the opinion of M. M. Foville and Bouillaud is supported by numerous cases ; still as there are some quite irreconcilable with it, we must examine further before we can determine what are the functions of the corpora striata and thalami.

PITUITARY BODY. — The brothers Wenzel, in investigating the pathology of epilepsy have found this body most frequently diseased of any part of the brain. In some cases it was much softer than natural, and in others firmer and greatly enlarged. Otto also noticed its morbid condition in epilepsy, but considered it rather accidental and thinks it might be either the cause or consequence of the disease. I recently found it much enlarged and

---

* Dictionnaire de Medecine et de Chirurgie Pratiques, Art. Encephale.
† Do.   do.   do.   Art. Encephalite

indurated in two cases of Delirium Tremens, that I examined with Dr. Gilman of New York.

PINEAL GLAND. — This has frequently been found diseased. Sometimes morbidly enlarged even to the size of an egg, and stony, sometimes enlarged and filled with fluid, but no particular symptoms have been attributed to disease of this part. In some cases when it has been found diseased, there was no mental disturbance.

The following is a case furnished by Sir G. Blane.

CASE XXII. — An officer aged 33, complained of slight pain and confusion of the head with impaired appetite. After ten weeks, nausea and pain in the eyeballs. He was then wounded in the head, lost much blood and the bone exfoliated, and he was much better for more than a year. Then headache, watchfulness, flushing, and opthalmia. Recovered after three months, but was never free from headache. It gradually increased ; was sometimes referred to a spot on the occiput, and sometimes through the whole head. Was much aggravated by motion, which produced a painful jarring in his head, and much increased by going to stool, pain at last excruciating, with numbness of the left hand, then sudden delirium, coma and death in three days, duration of the complaint, three years.

Morbid Appearances. — Three ounces of fluid in the ventricles, in the seat of the pineal gland, a little to the right side, a tumor the size of a nutmeg, internally it was like cheese, but organized. Ramollissement of the cerebellum.

M. Quesnay quotes a case given by M. Anel, of a soldier whose os frontis was fractured and a ball lodged in the brain. This person recovered, and the ball remained in his head for several years without disturbance of mind, and without producing any inconvenience. Finally while playing a game of cards, he died suddenly. On opening his head the ball was found lying upon the pineal gland, along with recently effused blood.

From these cases it seems the functions of this heretofore noted part of the brain, are not of great importance.

OPTIC TUBERCLES. — CORPORA QUADRIGEMINA. — Whenever these bodies are diseased, loss of sight ensues. Wenzel has noticed the wasting of the optic beds and Gall, that of the anterior tubercula quadrigemina in blind people. Wenzel has ascertained by minute researches, that in blindness, the optic beds first flatten, and then become narrower and shorter. " In long continued blindness of one eye," says Otto, "one of the optic beds is often wasted and generally that on the opposite, though also on the same side." In the *London Medical Gazette*, for Sept. 1838, Dr. Kerrison has recorded the following.

CASE XXIII. — A man aged 66, of temperate habits, had for three years been gradually losing his sight, and for two months had suffered from pain in the occipital region. When seen by Dr. Kerrison, April 23, he had complete amaurosis, with dilated and insensible pupil on the right side, and very indistinct vision (almost amounting to amaurosis) in the left eye. There was much dulness, and at the same time anxiety in his countenance; his mind was much confused; his answers sometimes rambling; and his utterance slow and heavy. His hearing and all his other senses were perfect. Under an antiphlogistic treatment with counter irritation to the back of the neck, his general health improved; but on the 8th May, he had a fit, and a second one on the 3d of June, on the 18th of June he became comatose, and died the afternoon of that day.

On examination, behind the third ventricle, and pressing on the corpora quadrigemina, and also partially on the cerebellum, there was a tumor the size of a walnut, of a cartilaginous nature, but which in some parts was soft and easily broken up. It was partly surrounded by a softish substance, having some points of bloody infiltration. This extended for some distance into the left hemisphere, on which side there was also about a drachm and a half of an amber colored gelatinous effusion lying over the choroid plexus, and in the posterior corner of the lateral ventricle.

CORPUS CALLOSUM. — The following case of a bullet lodged in the corpus callosum, is from Hennen.

CASE XXIV. — A soldier was shot in the head, and a fracture was the consequence, with a depression of not less than an inch and half, but, as no untoward symptom occurred, no operation was had recourse to. This man recovered, and went to the rear, where, at a distance of several weeks afterwards, he got an attack of phrenitis, from excessive drinking, and died. As the existence of the ball in the brain was strongly suspected, an inquiry was made after death, and, on dissection, it was found lodged in the corpus callosum.

FORNIX. — Andral says softening of the fornix occurs without producing any cerebral symptoms. The two following are from Abercrombie on Disease of the Brain.

CASE XXV. — A woman, aged 30, (18th June,) was affected with violent pain in the head, which extended across from temple to temple. She was extremly restless, owing to the intensity of the pain; eyes slightly effused, and impatient of light; pupils contracted; the pulse 60, soft and rather weak; tongue white. She was bled repeatedly, both generally and topically, and used

9*

purgatives, cold applications to the head, blistering, &c.
For three days she appeared much relieved ; the violent
pain was removed, and she complained of pain only
when she moved her head ; pulse from 80 to 90. She
was quite sensible, but considerably oppressed and inclined to lie without being disturbed. On the 22d, her
speech was affected ; she was sensible of it herself, and
said that " she felt a difficulty in getting out her words ; "
pulse 112. (23d and 24th.) Increasing stupor ; at times
incoherence, but, when roused, she answered questions
distinctly ; double vision ; made no complaint, but said her
head was better. Pulse from 112 to 120. (25th.) Increasing stupor. (26th.) Complete coma and dilated
pupil ; pulse 108, and of good strength ; died in the night.

Inspection. — The fornix and septum lucidum were
broken down into a soft white pulpy mass. There was
no other disease in any part of the brain.

CASE XXVI. — A man, aged 36, a blacksmith, had been
for some months affected with pectoral complaints, which
were considered as phthisical. On the 10th of November, 1818, being suddenly told of the death of his daughter, who died of phthisis, he suddenly complained of
headache ; and after another day or two, a remarkable
change was observed in his temper, which became uncommonly fretful and irascible. He still complained of
constant headache, which was much increased by motion ; his pulse varied from 70 to 110. In this state he
continued for a week, without any alleviation of the
headache. In the second week, he began to be slightly
delirious, with a tendency to stupor, the headache continuing very severe. He became gradually more and
more oppressed, and at last comatose ; and, after perfect
coma of four days' continuance, died on the 27th. His
pectoral symptoms had entirely subsided after the com-

mencement of the complaints in his head. I did not see this patient during his life, but was present at the examination of the body.

Inspection. — The membranes of the brain were very vascular. There was no effusion in the ventricles beyond the usual quantity. The septum lucidum was much broken down, and a large opening was formed through the centre of it. The fornix was reduced to a soft white mass, which could not be raised. There was no other morbid appearance in any part of the brain.

From these cases it would seem that neither the corpus callosum or fornix is concerned with the transmission of sensation or volition, as affections of these parts do not produce paralysis or derange sensation. How far they are connected with the intellectual powers seems undetermined, as in some cases related by Lallemand of disease of these parts, the mental powers were disturbed, while in those already alluded to, no intellectual derangement was observed. Probably the fornix and corpus callosum have nothing to do with the manifestations of the mental powers.

PONS VAROLII. — CRURA CEREBRI. — Solly says, " Lesions of these parts are almost invariably followed by paralysis of motion, but not always by that of sensation, a difference which appears to be connected simply with the extent of the disease. When inflammation first attacks one of the crura cerebri, it generally produces a tendency on the part of the patient to turn round ; if the inflammation continue its course uninterrupted, this is soon followed by hemiplegia."

The following is a case quoted by Lallemand from Bricheteau, of disease of the pons varolii.

CASE XXVII. — A woman, thirty-four years of age, had

been valetudinary for some time, and subject to wandering pains of the head, &c. On the 21st of March, 1816, she became, all at once, insensible, and continued in this state till the next day, when she was conveyed to the Hotel Dieu. She was then in a profound coma, the head thrown backwards, the eyes fixed and squinting, the pupils contracted and immovable, the members paralyzed and lying in any direction in which they were placed ; little or no sense of feeling, breathing slow and stertorous, temperature and pulse nearly natural. Sinapisms, emetics, &c., without any avail. Died two days afterward.

On dissection, the brain, except the tuber annulare, presented no trace of disease. The tuber was reduced to a sort of bouillie. The cerebellum was sound.

In the 12th volume of the *Lancet*, is related the case of a man who consulted Mr. Wardrop for pain of the head. Soon after, he complained of a want of power in his left arm and leg, and staggered in his walk. He also had difficulty of utterance, and finally lost the power of speech and the power of motion of both sides of the body. He continued in this state several days before he died, his intellect remaining undisturbed until his decease. On dissection, the principal disease was found in the pons varolii, which appeared as if lacerated, was extremely soft and pulpy, and on cutting into it was found to be converted into pultaceous matter, which could be washed away.

Mr. Yelloly has published in the first volume of the Medico Chirurgical Transactions, the following interesting case of disease of the same part of the brain.

CASE XXVIII.—David Thomas, a man of a fair complexion, and of about thirty-six years of age, became my patient in the General Dispensary, in December, 1806, on account of a slight paralysis of the right side, and a distortion of the left eye. He had been subject, for twelve months before, to occasional severe attacks of pain of the head, shooting from behind forwards; and about six weeks previous to my seeing him, he was surprised, on waking in the morning, to find his left eye drawn inwards, and his vision double. In two or three days more, his right hand became weak; and this was gradually followed by weakness, and afterwards by numbness of the corresponding side; and by a slight stammering, and a small degree of distortion of the mouth.

These symptoms continued when I first saw him, with some degree of headache, and his pulse about sixty-eight, and rather weaker in the affected than the sound arm. In other respects, he was in his accustomed state of health. The left eye was drawn towards the nose, but the pupil was in its usual state of sensibility to light. The double vision continued. All voluntary power over the abductor muscle was lost; nor did the affected eye, as in common cases of strabismus, recover its usual position on shutting the sound one. He had been purged and blistered by a gentleman well versed in the treatment of complaints of the eye, when the distortion first came on; but he ceased to be under his care on the paralysis supervening.

In little more than a week from the time of my first seeing him, he became at first slightly, and then considerably affected with convulsive motions of the whole body. These recurred at more and more frequent intervals, he became gradually less and less sensible, and died in about twenty-four hours from their commencement. I saw him a few hours previous to his death. He was then in a state of insensibility, with his eyes suffused, his pulse weak, frequent, and fluttering, and his respiration laborious. The distorted eye had recovered its usual position a few hours before, and the pupils were insensible to the action of light.

On dissection, the brain was found to be of an unusually firm texture, with about half an ounce of water in the ventricles. There was no deceased appearance in the right side of the head, but in the left, a tumor was discovered on the tuberculum annulare, which my friend and colleague, Mr. Thomas Blizard, surgeon to the London Hospital, did me the favor to examine with me. It was about the size of a hazel nut, and was lying on, and sunk into the terberculum, at its posterior part, on the left side. It extended to the corpus pyramidale of the same side, pressing upon, and entirely obscuring the left abductor nerve.

The following case from the Archives Generales, 1834, is worthy of notice.

CASE XXIX. — "A middle-aged man was lately admitted into the Hotel Dieu. The symptoms were feverishness, great debility, confusion of head, and inability to use his limbs, at least freely. There was no abdominal or pectoral distress. When he was put to bed, it was observed that the head was in a state of continual rotation, even when resting upon the pillow ; it was not bent forwards or backwards, but only rolled about from side to side ; the muscles of the face were occasionally convulsed, but the mouth was not distorted, nor was the tongue drawn either to the right or the left side, although constantly moving with a tremulous agitation. Both forearms exhibited a prolonged convulsive movement along their radial sides, so that the thumbs and fore-fingers were kept bent ; the soles of the feet were turned inwards and upwards ; the tendons of the tibialis antici muscles were very prominent, and permanently stiff. The patient seemed to have a complete control over the flexors and extensors of the head ; when assisted, he could raise himself up and sit in bed.   The movements of the thoracic and abdominal muscles were healthy. The voluntary movements of the extremities were very imperfect ; he could not raise his left arm at all to his head, and his right one only with considerable difficulty. The common sensibility was but little affected in any part ; the intellect was confused ; he could not answer many questions successively.   In the course of a few days, all the unfavorable symptoms were agravated ; the trembling oscillation of the head and tongue were incessant ; the trunk and limbs lay nearly still and motionless ; the forearms were laid across the abdomen, the wrists were bent, and the thumbs drawn into the hollow of the hand, and almost constantly trembling.   Every now and then there was a paroxysm of apparently epileptic convulsions, and the patient seemed to recover his sensibility and consciousness for a time, but he soon relapsed into his former stupor.   On dissection, the attention of the physician was directed in a special manner to the encephalic contents ; and it was found that a tumor, of the size of a small walnut, had formed on the tuber annulare, and adhered to the outer surface of the cerebellum. This tumor was formed of nacreous particles and layers, and belonged to that class of morbid deposits described by M. Cruveilhier as consisting of stearine and cholesterine ; they appear to be quite inorganic, presenting no traces of vessels, or of cellular tissue."

Some of the symptoms witnessed in the foregoing cases were probably caused by pressure upon the surrounding parts, still it is evident from them that the pons varolii is not concerned in the operations of the intellect.

Let us now inquire if pathology has afforded us any

further knowledge of the functions of the different parts of the brain.

In medical writings, we find numerous cases of loss or derangement of some particular faculties of the mind, arising from disease or injury of the brain, while other faculties do not appear to be disturbed. We will here particularize some of the most remarkable of these.

First. — In the 30th volume of the *Edinburgh Medical and Surgical Journal,* is a very interesting case, or would be if the appearances on dissection were more fully given. It was the case of a woman who had a tumor on the forehead the size of an egg, which subjected her to severe headache and epileptic fits, which finally caused her death. On dissection, a small abscess was found in the right anterior lobe of the brain, and an osseous tumor in the left, thus disorganizing both anterior lobes. The history of the case, so far as relates to the mental powers, was, that after the commencement of the tumor, her temper changed ; from being mild in disposition, she became very irascible. Her intellect also suffered. She lost the power of adding numbers. She forgot the looks of her most intimate friends, but seemed to recognize them by the voice. She also lost the power of discriminating colors, and of recollecting names. She retained her taste for music, and appeared at times religiously insane, and always went to church.

Second. — Rochoux (Recherches sur l'Apoplexie, Paris, 1814,) relates that a man from a blow on his head, became embarrassed in speech, to which succeeded coma and death. On dissection, a tumor filled with blood, and of the size of an egg, was found in the anterior part of the left hemisphere of the brain.

Third. — Andral (Clinique Medicale,) relates a similar case of a tumor in the same situation producing extreme difficulty in pronouncing words. After articulating with great difficulty some few words, there was nothing heard but one unmeaning stammering.

Fourth. — Hennen, in his Principles of Military Surgery, has given an interesting case, of which the following is an abridgement.

CASE XXX. — Captain B——, a particular friend of mine, was wounded by a musket ball in the head, at Waterloo, on the 18th of June, 1815. On the 19th, he was brought into the city of Brussels, in charge of a medical officer, who gave me a most melancholy account of his case. On approaching the wagon in which he was conveyed, I was insensibly attracted to that part of it where he was stretched, by a low protracted moan, as of a person in extreme pain, but very weak. On calling him by name, he sat up, caught me by the hand, which he kissed most fevently, pointed to his head, and then to the site of a former wound, which he had received at the storming of Badajoz, in 1812, from the effects of which I had the good fortune to relieve him. He then burst into tears, but without having the power of uttering a distinct word. His countenance was pale and ghastly, and his mouth somewhat distorted ; his eye languid, and suffused with blood ; his skin dry, but cool ; his pulse about 90, soft and compressible.

On examining the wound of the head, I found an extensive radiated fracture, occupying almost the whole of the left parietal bone ; at the centre, there was a piece of bone apparently the size of a musket ball, beat in through the membranes of the brain, and bedded in its substance, but considerably more toward the frontal region than the occipital. The unequal pressure I found to proceed from a musket ball, which was wedged in between the displaced pieces of bone and the portion

10

which, though cracked, preserved its situation. The separate piece was obviously much more extensive on its internal face than externally, and could not possibly be extracted without the operation of trephining, to which I proceeded. The leaden wedge, and several loose splinters which jammed it in, were easily removed; and on making one perforation with a large sized trephine, I removed the depressed portion of bone, which was forced into the brain nearly an inch and a half from the surface of the scalp. It was of an irregularly oval shape, about one inch long by half an inch broad, and fractured in such a manner, that the internal table formed a much larger part of its circumference than the external.

No relief followed the operation; he passed an extremely restless night, and the pulse rose so rapidly and so high, that the abstraction of 16 ounces of blood became necessary. But the next day a spontaneous bilious diarrhœa came on, and he was much more sensible. He made an attempt to articulate, and pronounced audibly the letter T, once or twice. The next morning, being the fifth from the receipt of the wound, his general appearance was amazingly altered for the better; the diarrhœa still remained, and his efforts to speak were continued. On the sixth day, he grasped my hand with great fervor, looked pitiously in my face, and to my inquiries as to his feelings, he uttered audibly, though with much labor, the monosylable, "THER," to which, in the course of the day he added " O !" and for the next three days, whenever addressed, he slowly, distinctly, and in a most pathetic tone, repeated the words, " O ! THER ; O ! THER," as if to prove his powers of pronunciation. His general appearance during all this time, amended considerably, and my hopes now began to revive. I therefore resolved to write to his family, and, before doing so,

I printed in large characters, on a sheet of paper, the following words, "SHALL I WRITE TO YOUR MOTHER?" that being the wish which it appeared to me he so long and ardently had labored to utter. It is impossible to describe the illumination of his countenance on reading these talismanic words; he grasped and pressed my hand with warmth, burst into tears, and gave every demonstration of having obtained the boon which he had endeavored to solicit.

From this period his mental faculties gradually developed themselves; he regained a consciousness of the circumstances immediately preceding his wound, and, in succession, of those of a more remote period. The power of speech was the last which he perfectly regained, and for which he usually substituted the communication of his thoughts and wishes in writing. Throughout the whole of his convalescent state, melancholy ideas constantly predominated, although, previous to the accident, he had been remarkable for his flow of spirits. He returned to England, nearly recovered, on the 29th of September, or 103d day from the wound.

This case may be advantageously compared with one given by M. Larrey,* in which a soldier, wounded in the head, formed a new language for himself. He expressed affirmation not by "Oui," but by the word "Baba." Negatives he gave by "Lala;" and his wants he made known by the terms "Dada" and "Tata." These sounds bore no analogy to the words properly expressive of his ideas. Captain B., on the contrary, strenuously labored to combine all the simple sounds which composed the words that he wished to express.

Fifth.—Larrey's case referred to above, was that of

---

*Memoirs, vol. iii, p. 322.

a soldier wounded by a ball, in the left temple, near the orbit. He died three months after the accident, of fever, and on examining his head, portions of the convolutions at the anterior part of the brain were found to be effaced, and the dura mater thickened.

Sixth. — In the celebrated case of Dupuytren, in which, in search of an abscess, he plunged a bistory above an inch into the substance of the brain, through a hole made by the trephine, in the right parietal bone, the patient was instantly deprived of the power of speech.

Seventh. — In the *Lancette Francaise*, 1833, is a case of an officer wounded by a ball in the right frontal sinus. Amaurosis and a total loss of the memory of events and objects, was the consequence.

Eighth. — Dr. Adair Crawford says, " We remember an interesting case under the care of Dr. Cuming of Armagh, in which there was disease in the anterior part of the brain, from a blow received on the forehead, just above the nose; it was found necessary to remove a portion of the bone with a trephine ; and after a variety of remarkable and untoward symptoms, the gentleman recovered ; one of the prominent symptoms was a loss of the memory of language.*

M. Bouillaud states that disorganization of the anterior lobes of the brain, causes loss of speech, either from the loss of the memory of words, or the loss of the power of muscular motion of the organs of speech. He thinks that disorder of the grey substance of the anterior lobes produces the loss of the memory of words — of all that is intellectual in speech, while injury of the white portion of the anterior lobes, produces an impossibility of conducting the movements necessary to articulate.

---

*Cyclopedia Practical Medicine.   Art. Inflammation of the Brain.

Many more cases might be adduced of the loss of particular mental faculties from injury and disease of the brain, but for the most part they are so carelessly and imperfectly given, that it is impossible to make out what part of the brain was affected.

It is much to be regretted the skull has not been divided into regions, so that descriptions of its injuries could be rendered more clear and exact. Many writers content themselves with stating that the wound was on the forehead, or vertex, or on the left or right side. These terms do not enable us to know the precise situation of the injury. The phrenological chart might perhaps be useful to correct this evil, if the location of the organs was the same in all. And at present it may be serviceable to aid us in understanding the place of injury.

I recommend the following division of the skull. Let a line from the root of the nose to the middle of the back of the neck, corresponding to the longitudinal sinus, be called the *median line*. Let another from the meatus externus of one side be extended over the head to the other, called the *transverse line*. Then describe the injuries of the skull in reference to these lines, by inches and parts of inches.

For example, the precise situation of a wound would be made known, if said to be on the right or left side, and an inch and a half anterior to the transverse line, and an inch from the median. Its situation might, in some cases, be better understood by referring to other marked points on the head, as the eyebrows, and their angles.

From the preceding notice of the various methods of studying the functions of the brain, we perceive that pathological investigations have contributed the most to extend our knowledge of these functions. From this source, we have learned,

First. — That the cerebral lobes, or the hemispheres of the cerebrum, are the seat of intelligence.

Second. — That the cincritious portion of these lobes, probably, is, the seat of the mental faculties.

Third. — That the fibrous or medullary portions of the brain are connected with the motive powers, and transmit volition and sensation.

Fourth. — That the lobes of the cerebellum are not connected with the manifestations of the mental powers, but are with the motive; and appear also to be with the sexual propensity, and that the sympathy between them and the stomach is intimate.

Fifth. — That all the faculties of the mind may be manifested by one hemisphere of the brain.

Sixth. — That different parts of the brain have different functions, and that the anterior portion of the cerebral lobes play the most important part in manifesting the mental powers, and appear to be the seat of the memory of words, events, and numbers

Seventh. — That the striated bodies and the thalami are intimately associated with the motive powers of the extremities.

Eighth. — That parts in the middle and at the base of the brain, such as the fornix, corpus callosum, septum lucidum, pituitary body, and pineal gland, are not connected with the mental faculties.

We thus see how useful pathological investigations have been; we also see that the field of inquiry is still very great, and that numerous researches are nesessary to enable us to understand the functions of all the parts of the brain.

But what we have learned by this method of inquiry, should induce us to persevere; to examine with care every disease of the brain and to learn and record its history and all the symptoms by which it is accompanied.

As an *example* of this method of investigating the functions and diseases of the brain and nervous system, I know not of any more worthy of being followed, than that adopted by Dr. Bright, as will be seen by the following cases and remarks published by him in Guy's Hospital Reports, for April 1837, and which I select from the Medico Chirurgical Review, for July 1837.

CASE XXXI. — " In Nov. 1831, Dr. Bright was sent for to Woolwich, to see an officer, a tall athletic man, aged 48, who, after being many years in active foreign service, had returned home in 1817. He married in 1825, and had a family. In 1826, he suffered severely from sciatica of the right hip, which he had injured some years before, by a fall from his horse. This was cured by carbonate of iron ; and he afterwards enjoyed an excellent state of health, till the autum of 1829, when being again engaged in foreign service, he began to experience an attack of periodic pain over the left eye, exactly in the superorbitar notch. This pain used to return about dinnertime, daily ; and was always put a stop to, before he had half finished his meal. At this time he met with a very severe accident ; and was taken up, stunned, and senseless. He was bled ; and, after some hours, recovered ; but his recollection was, for a day or two, so defective, that he frequently asked what service they were engaged in, and what they were doing ; and it was with great difficulty these points could be explained to him. However, in a short time he was tolerably restored ; though he never regained the state of health he had enjoyed before his fall, frequently complained of pains in his head, and of some weakness in his right leg.

" About Christmas, he had a severe attack of bilious vomiting; after which, the pains in his head, and over the right eye, were worse, and more frequent; and he experienced, occasionally, a temporary loss of sight, coming over him like a cloud, and lasting for some minutes; then passing off, and not being followed by any remarkable increase of the headache. After some weeks of suffering, the intermittent pain over the left eye was completely removed in a single day, by taking three doses of sulphate of quinine in rapid succession, two or three hours before the expected diurnal attack; and it never afterwards returned. In June, 1830, he had another attack of bilious vomiting, of great severity; which however, passed off so quickly, that the following day he was able to resume all his duties; but shortly afterwards he discovered, one morning, that the sight of the left eye was completely gone. The sight of the right eye also became imperfect; the weakness of the right leg increased; and the left leg also began to lose power. In 1831, when he returned home, the sight of one eye was entirely lost; and with the other, it was only by great effort, and by changing the field of vision often, that he could discover the features of any one with whom he conversed. The hearing of the right ear was tolerably perfect; but he had, for many years, lost the hearing of the left, from the shock of a gun firing. He likewise complained much of pain darting through his head; which was relieved by cupping, blistering, and tar-tar-emetic ointment.

" Dr. B. first saw him on the 8th Nov. 1831. He was then sitting in his chair, perfectly unconscious of surrounding objects, nor was he aware of Dr. Bright's presence. When, after much trouble, by writing words on his hand and by calling in his ear, and by other means, he was led

to comprehend, he answered distinctly, and without hesitation, but in the high-raised, and ill-modulated voice
which is usually observed in deaf people. His intellect
seemed unimpaired. He was able to stand ; but, partly
from the weakness of his lower extremities, and still more
from the timidity arising from his blindness, he could not
move without support ; and when he attempted to walk,
it was with a short, feeble, tottering step. He had no
incontinence of urine, although that had occasionally appeared some weeks before ; he had never passed his fæces unconsciously, but once or twice there had scarcely
been time to prevent an accident of that kind. His sleep
was tranquil, and not too heavy ; nor did he appear more
drowsy than might be expected in a person deprived of
sight and hearing. His appetite was good, and had sometimes been excessive. There was some inequality in his
power of hearing. At times he could catch sounds, but
never distinctly, as to understand their meanings. About
a week before Dr. B's visit, he had had a fit, with temporary insensibility and suffused countenance, but without convulsion.

"In the course of November, he partially recovered
his hearing, being able once or twice to distinguish the
drum or the bugle sounding, nay, even certain words.
If made to hear what was said, he comprehended it and
answered rightly. Dr. B. again saw him on the 29th.
He had sometimes spoken of a very peculiar sensation in
his head, attended with a sound as if grease had been
thrown into the fire, making a whizzing noise, and then
dying away, whilst at the same time a flash of light passed over his eyes. His sight had also been occasionally
improved. He was strong on his legs. The pulse varied from 70 to 75. Light bitters with the volatile alkali,
blisters, and a seton were the means employed.

"After this, the symptoms gradually increased, and

the mental faculties grew weaker.   Dr. B. saw him again on the 14th of November, 1832.   He was then in bed, helpless, and much emaciated.   His wife was feeding him with meat, finely minced, and mixed with potatoes ; she was obliged to rouse him frequently, to make him take his food ; and then he continued to open and close his teeth gently, till he fell asleep, while the meat still remained partly in his mouth.   Taste appeared to be lost. He was quite unconscious, and usually in a kind of slumber, but, on some days, was more drowsy than on others. If conscious of the calls of nature, he gave no intimation that he was so.   The pupils seemed quite motionless. He occasionally expressed severe headache, and a pain over the right eye.

" He died on the 27th of December.   He had sunk progressively, and sloughs formed on the sacrum before death.

" *Dissection.* — The scalp rather more bloodless than usual.   The skull was hard and solid, and somewhat uneven in its thickness : on each side of the sagittal suture internally, but particularly on the left, it had small, deep, irregular cavities, which had been filled with corresponding unusually enlarged glandulæ Pacchioni, which seemed to have almost perforated the skull in some parts, so that only the external table remained.   The dura mater was not very vascular ; but the projection of the glandular bodies, on each side of the longitudinal sinus, was remarkable ; so that, at first, they suggested the idea of small cerebriform fungous tumors.   A small bony plate also, about half an inch in length, lay along the angle of the falx.   The longitudinal sinus was quite natural.   The dura mater adhered very firmly to the arachnoid, at those parts where the glands were so large ; and when it was removed, the arachnoid in the immediate neighborhood was white and opaque.   The arachnoid was not vascular, nor unnaturally adherent to the brain. There was no serum effused beneath it. The depth between the two hemispheres of the cerebrum was small, owing to a considerable elevation of the corpus callosum. The general substance of the brain was natural, but rather deficient in bloody points.

" The roof of the ventricles was raised high by clear fluid, of which about four ounces were collected, both the posterior and anterior portion of the ventricles being distended : but the accumulation appeared greatest in the anterior. A few large vessels, ramified on the internal surfaces of the ventricles, the corpora striata, and the optic thalami, seemed flattened ; and the septum lucidum was much thicker and firmer than natural. The choroid plexus, on each side, was exsanguine, and contained several vesicles, from the size of a pin's head to that of a pea. The velum interpositum was also exsanguine.

" In attempting to remove the brain from the basis of the skull, it was found that the anterior portion of the cerebellum, on the left side, degenerated into a tumor ; and adhered so firmly, that it could not be detached without a scalpel, or employing considerable force, from the petrous portion of the temporal bone. The structure of this tumor was chiefly hard and unyielding, but in some parts softer ; and the nervus trigeminus, or fifth nerve, was seen passing over it, flattened and broad ; nor did the tumor simply adhere, but the bone had become carious, and pervaded by it, so that a softened cavity occupied a large portion of the petrous ridge, extending towards the sella turcica."

CASE XXXII. — " N. Wells, aged 43, admitted into Guy's Hospital, October 22d, 1834.

" In 1817, he received a wound from the bursting of a gun, by which his cheek bone was much injured, and which was followed by defective hearing in the left ear. No other ill consequences followed until 18 months ago, when an offensive discharge took place from the left ear, which, after continuing for eight months, suddenly stopped about Christmas last. This was quickly followed by a pain across the forehead, and a sense of weight towards the back of the head. About four months ago, the vision of the left eye became imperfect; and in another month, the right eye was likewise affected.

" At the time of his admission, the vision of both eyes had, for the last month been so defective, that he was unable to find his way in the street. During the last six weeks, he had been attacked, three or four times almost every day, with a convulsive agitation, chiefly affecting the left side; and he stated that his memory had become very imperfect respecting recent circumstances, but was more retentive of those of earlier date. His pulse was variable in strength and frequency, generally about 96.

" He remained under Dr. Bright's care for nearly three months. The treatment consisted in calomel, leeches, counter-irritation, &c.,; but it was of no service. The chief variations which took place, during the time he remained, were the occasional recurrence of very severe headaches. He once or twice fell to the ground, in fits of giddiness; and was often unable to move, from what he called the heaviness of his head. He had occasional difficulty in passing his urine; and his bowels were costive. On the 13th of January, he left the hospital, being at that time totally blind; and never afterwards could distinguish light from darkness. He was quite deaf in the left ear, and the hearing of the right was at times .much affected. He had then the perfect use of his limbs; and was in the habit of being led out for walks to a considerable distance. In this state he continued until the Summer of 1835, when he was suddenly attacked one day while walking, and fell insensible. He was attended by Mr. Griffith, a very intelligent surgeon, of Pimlico, who reports that after this ; —

" He was hemiplegic on the right side, and the mouth was drawn to the left. On the side affected, there was total loss of sensation. He recovered, in some degree, sensation, and the power of motion in the arm and leg ; but the effort to use either was always accompanied with violent shaking. He could not stand without support. He at all times had the power of retaining and voiding his fæces and urine ; the bowels were very torpid, requiring the daily use of full doses of aperient medicine to procure relief. He was subject to convulsive attacks : which came on sometimes three times, sometimes only once a day, and sometimes with an intermission of a day or two. His mind was at times childish, but his reason was not gone ; his sense of taste was entirely destroyed ; his hearing varied, being sometimes very good, at others imperfect. Though I had not seen him for many months he immediately recognised me by my voice. This was about two months before his death ; he then articulated with much difficulty ; he uttered his words suddenly, and after a prolonged effort. His tongue was drawn forcibly to the roof of his mouth ; and in the effort to speak, there was apparently great difficulty to depress the lower jaw ; he frequently, however, gaped, and yawned to the full extent. It appeared that the muscles of the right side of the jaw had in. a degree regained their power ; for the distortion, when I saw him, was in no great degree : sensation, however, was entirely lost on this side of the face. He was a man of irritable temper, and passionate ; but I did not observe that he was lately more so than usual. For a considerable time before his death, his arms were so paralyzed, that he could not feed himself ; and for the last ten weeks, he could not

11

leave his bed on account of the paralyzed state of his legs."

" He died on the 24th of October, 1836, and was examined by Mr. Griffith, in the presence of Mr. Dewsnap, Mr. Bowling, and Dr. Bright.

"*Dissection.* — On raising the calvaria, the dura mater appeared tense, but not remarkably vascular. Two or three large glandulæ Pacchioni stood out on its surface, by the side of the longitudinal sinus, like little fungoid excrescences. When the dura mater was removed the convolutions appeared flattened, from the profusion of fluid in the ventricles. The arachnoid was not very vascular, and there was no serious effusion.

" On cutting into the substance of the brain, there was decided marks of congestion internally, and very distinct mottling. The corpus callossum was a little raised. The ventricles were distended to three times their natural size, by limpid fluid ; the parietes and septum lucidum were firm ; the foramen of Monro was large and open ; one large vessel ran meandering along the under edge of the plexus choroides ; the plexus itself was exsanguine.

" The optic nerves were remarkably small, hard, and of a yellow color, very different from the pure white by which they are usually distinguished. Their section was oval and compressed. The infundibulum was rather thicker, and of firmer consistence than natural.

" Beneath the tentorium, a tumor, as large as a chesnut, was found on the left side, apparently attached by a peduncle to the petrous portion of the temporal bone, pushing aside the tuber annulare and the left hemisphere of the cerebellum, compressing the medulla oblongata, and pushing the fifth nerve upwards. This was found to be a firm dark tumor, the section of which was mottled with grumous blood ; and it altogether bore the appearance of a fungoid growth, arising from the cancellated structure of the bone, but closely attached to the anterior portion of the cerebellum. The cancelli of the bone were soft, containing a puriform fluid. The tympanum was quite gone ; and the ear contained some purulent matter.

" In the lower part of the thorax, on the left side, was a circumscribed chronic empyema, of some standing.

" The following observations by Dr. Bright are a good example of rational and supported generalization. It would be well, if all other observations in medicine were as rational and as supported.

" In both cases, we have individuals, little past the prime of life, dying in consequence of tumors similarly situated within the skull ; and, as they were both in other respects healthy, their symptoms had suffered no important complications from the co-existence of other diseases. In both, we have reason to connect the aggravation and probably the existence of the disease with the exposures and accidents of military service. In both, the disease has been marked by its gradual progress ; has first shown itself by affections of the senses ; and then slowly produced paralysis of motion or sensation in various parts, affecting the intellect little, until an advanced period of the disease, and probably not before it had led to extensive serious effusion into the ventricles.

" The symptoms may be more specifically stated ; as, an almost total loss of sight, total loss of hearing in one ear, and to a great extent in both, gradual paralysis of the extremities, slight and temporary affection of the sphincters, great diminution in the sense of taste, and a protracted death from sensorial oppression.

" In these two cases, the left ear lost its sensibility not much less than twenty years before death ; in the one, from the concussion of a cannon ; in the other, after a severe wound in the face, and, doubtless, concussion of the temporal bone. What predisposing influence was exercised by the violence inflicted at that time, in either case, it is impossible to say; but the circumstances should not be lost sight of, in the record of facts.

" In both cases the vision was impaired and destroyed, even before the hearing of the right ear; and it is not easy to account for this affection of the sight. I am sorry that I cannot find any observation after death on the condition of the optic nerves in the first case; and I therefore suppose that no remarkable change was observable in their appearance, or that it was passed over unobserved. In the second case a very obvious alteration presented itself, the nerves being small, hard, and dark colored, with a yellow tint, and, to all appearance, unfitted for the discharge of their natural function; but how this change was induced, whether by pressure on any part of their course, or by interruption to the circulation through their substance, or by the irritation of contiguous parts, or in consequence of the serous effusion taking place in the ventricles, I do not pretend to say. The loss of vision, in both cases, leads us to suppose that it forms an important part of the consecutive history of the disease. The loss of sight in the left eye took place, in each, rather more than two years before death; and the loss of vision in the right eye followed very shortly after that in the left. The left ear, though its power was diminished to a very great extent in both cases, and was entirely lost in the first, retained its faculty of receiving impressions longer than either of the eyes.

"The situation of the organic mischief, which might be said, in both cases, to encroach upon the mechanism of the right ear, and which made pressure on the auditory nerve of that side, afforded sufficient explanation of the destruction of its functions; but it is probably to the pressure communicated, through the pons Varolii, to the auditory nerve on the opposite side, as the tumors enlarged, that we may ascribe the slow diminution of sense in the left ear.

"With regard to the sense of taste, it seems to have been impaired, in the case, as each disease gradually advanced ; and in neither is any specific notice taken of it, till a few months before death. This is one of the most peculiar and interesting symptoms because one of the least frequently noticed in cases of cerebral lesion ; and I have no doubt that it arose from pressure made by the tumor of the fifth pair of nerves, which gives origin to the gustatory branch ; for, in both cases, the fifth pair suffered the most obvious and decided displacement and compression. The obtuseness of the sense displaced itself in the total want of preference with respect to articles taken into the mouth, as observed in the first case, so that the most nauseous medicines were taken with the same indifference as the most grateful beverages ; and, in the second case, the inability to distinguish flavors was freely admitted."

We occasionally see disease of the brain, that appears to disorder but one faculty of the mind, producing what is called monomonia. Such instances deserve very careful investigation. The following is an important case published by Dr. Scott, of Cupar, Fife.

CASE XXXIII. — " The subject was a navy surgeon, (John Anderson, M. D.) who being placed with many others on half-pay, after the downfall of Napolean, came to reside in his native town of Cupar. His manners and acquirements caused his society to be courted ; but, as he tried several times to settle in practice, and was always disappointed, he became liable to fits of despondency. In 1820, five years after his discharge from the

11*

public service, his eccentricities of thought, especially on one particular subject, were remarked by his friends. He had been diving into the mysteries, not to say the absurdities of animal magnetism, and at last became convinced that he himself was subject to its powerful influence, exerted by some of his best friends. He now became sleepless; or, if he slept, he was the victim of those " terrors magici," conjured up by oppressive and phantastic dreams. Certain individuals could wield at will a malignant influence over him, so as to deprive him of all rest and enjoyment. To escape these *invisibles*, as he termed them, he went to Paris, in the year 1822, but his magnetic enemies soon mingled with the gay crowds on the Boulevards ! In the night these inexorable fiends would press on his breast with the weight of a millstone, disturbing his sleep and locking up his bowels : At other times, they directed their evil influence to the bladder or rectum, so that he would not have time to undress himself before their contents were discharged. On some occasions, these tormenters would take such unwarrantable liberties with him that he was found to roar aloud ; and, several times he applied to the local authorities for protection. On all other subjects he was perfectly sane, on this point he was decidedly mad. In process of time however, he began to evince symptoms of something more than imaginary hallucination. His memory in some particular points, failed him. He had the ideas apparently in his mind, but he could not clothe them in words. Having experienced several attacks of pneumonia, he became subject, for several months before he died, to a short dry cough, with severe pain in the back, oppression and tightness across the chest. On the day of his death, he had invited some friends to dine with him; but just as they were sitting down to the repast, their host began to cough up large quantities of blood, and in a few minutes, he died suffocated.

Dissection. — There was a large aneurism of the descending thoracic aorta, shewing the usual fibrinous matter, in concentric layers, which had pressed upon the roots of the bronchia, and eroded some of the dorsal vertebræ. This aneurism had burst into the trachea, and thus caused sudden death. In the head there was found an inflammatory deposite, apparently of long standing, under the arachnoid coat, with thickening of the membrane itself, and adhesion to the parts beneath, about the space of an inch and a half in length, and one in breadth, on each side of the longitudinal sinus, midway between the *crista galli*, and the level of the commencement of the lateral sinuses. No other change of structure could be detected."

Here was a case of monomania, or mental derangement on only one subject, and dissection showed very slight disease, and that confined to one portion of the brain. Like examinations of the brain after death, from other varieties of monomania, are much to be desired. Opportunities are not very rare. We often see cases of loss of the memory of words, of places, &c., without other mental disturbance. Among the inmates of lunatic hospitals, we frequently find patients maniacal but on one subject. I recently saw a female — a mother, who exhibited no other mental derangement than the total loss of the memory of her children, and of all affection for them. Every case of monomania deserves the most careful study during life, and after death, the brain should be minutely examined, and the whole history of the disease and appearances on dissection, be faithfully reported. In this manner much may in a few years be added to our knowledge of the functions of the most important, and, at present, least perfectly understood, organ of the body.

7. *External Examination of the Cranium. — Phrenology.*

Dr. Gall should be considered the first who directed attention to this method of studying the functions of the brain.* Many, I am aware, have condemned and ridiculed this method, but it appears to me eminently deserving of attention. One of the most distinguished of modern philosophers and metaphysicians observes, "There seems to be but little doubt, that *general* inferences concerning the intellectual capacity, may be drawn with some confidence from the form and the size of the skull, and it has been imagined by some, that corresponding to the varieties of intellectual and moral character, there are certain inequalities or prominences on the surface of the skull; *and it certainly is a legitimate object of experimental inquiry to ascertain how far this opinion is agreeable to fact.*"† With such high authority in favor of thus investigating the functions of the brain, surely we should not deem this method unworthy of our notice. For my own part, I see nothing unreasonable or unphilosophical in it, but can say in the language of one of the most celebrated of modern anatomists, that "the whole subject of phrenology appears to me of far too much importance to be discussed without the most rigid and impartial examination of the immense body of facts adduced in support of it; and this I have not hitherto had leisure to

* See Dr. Gall's great work, "On the Functions of the Brain and of each of its parts." Also the Phrenological works of Spurzheim and Combe.

† Dugald Stewart on Natural Language.

undertake. I shall therefore only say that, so far as I am acquainted with the subject, I do not see it as otherwise than rational and perfectly consistent with all that is known of the functions of the nervous system."*

It appears to me that Dr. Gall proceeded in a philosophical and cautious manner in forming his system, and that he is entitled to the praise of fairness and candor, as well as that of unsurpassed industry. He acknowledges the difficulties of the subject, and declares that, " to speak correctly of organology and cranioscopy, it is necessary to acquire a knowledge of it by a long and practical study." He fully notices the objections brought against his system ; indeed, he was the first to state these objections, and that in certain cases the external table of the cranium is not parallel to the inner one, that sometimes the crania of men of very limited capacity are exceedingly thick, even when this condition is not the result of advanced age or mental disease, both of which produce variations in the thickness of the cranium, and he declares that it is impossible to determine with exactness the developements of certain convolutions by the inspection of the external surface of the cranium. Besides, Dr. Gall never pretended that he was able to determine the character of men in general by the external examination of the head. " I have never pretended," says he, " to distinguish the influence, which modifications of the forms of the cranium slightly marked, may have on the character, or how its corresponding shades may be traced. My first observations have only been made upon persons who were distinguished from other men, by some eminent quality or faculty. I easily perceived that it was only in such individuals, that I could find striking differences of the head, and that I could dis-

* Solly, on the Human Brain, p. 471.

tinguish well marked protuberences."* Since the an-
nouncement of Dr. Gall's opinions, there have been many
discoveries in physiology, and numerous pathological researches bearing upon the functions of the nervous system.   These have not shaken the system of Gall, but on
the whole, have strengthened it.   In fact, I am confident
that opinions respecting the brain being a congeries of
organs exercising different functions, and the probability
of learning something respecting the functions of the
brain by the external examination of the skull, would
have been by this time advanced and embraced by many,
solely in consequence of the physiological and pathological discoveries and researches to which I have alluded.

So far as regards my personal observation on this subject, I am compelled to say, it has not been great.   The
attention I have given to it, has, however, impressed me
favorably   I have never found any striking instances in
contradiction of what Dr. Gall considers established.
For three years I have been a Director of the Connecticut
State Prison, and have had abundant opportunity of examining and comparing the heads and learning the character of several hundreds of prisoners.   I have not, to
be sure, embraced the opportunity thus afforded of studying this subject as thoroughly as I might.   Still, I have
not been wholly neglectful of it, and can state that I have
found, in numerous instances, confirmation of the opinions of Gall.

In conclusion, I consider this method of studying the
functions of the brain deserving of the attention of medical men, who, of all others, have the best opportunity of
testing its correctness and determining its value, particularly by pathological investigations.

---

* Gall, on the Functions of the Brain and each of its parts, &c.,
vol. 3.

SECTION III.

DISEASES AND FUNCTIONS OF THE MEDULLA OBLONGATA, AND MEDULLA SPINALIS.

By the medulla oblongata, I mean the upper or cranial portion of the spinal cord, that portion of it which lies within the cranium, extending from the pons varolii to the occipatal foramen. It is considerably larger than the spinal cord, and its functions more important. This enlargement seems to arise principally from deposites of cineriteous matter in seperate masses, which form four projections, two on each side. Thus, the medulla oblongata is made up of medullary fibrous columns, for the transmission of sensation and volition, and of these deposites of cineritious matter, the latter constiuting the difference between the medulla oblongata and the spinal cord. " The view," says Solly, " I am inclined to take of the character of the parts comprising the medulla oblongata is simply this : in addition to the columns for motion and sensation, there are here deposited, and imbedded to a certain extent in its substance, four ganglia, two on each side. The most anterior of these are the ovoid bodies, which derive the name of *olivary* from their form ; they seem to me to be the appropriate ganglia of the pneumo-gastric nerves.

" The posterior ganglia are found in the fissure at the back part of the cord, which is known by the absurd name of fourth ventricle. They form two projections of a pyramidal figure, and are usually designated the *posterior pyramidal bodies.* In these bodies terminate the auditory or eighth pair of nerves."

On each side of the anterior fissure of the medulla

oblongata, are other eminences, called the anterior pyramidal bodies, or *corpora pyramidalia ;* these are not occasioned by deposites of cineriteous matter, but by the
crossing over of the fibres of the anterior columns from
one-side to the other, a peculiarity of much importance,
and to which we shall again allude.

The functions of the medulla oblongata have been
greatly exalted by many physiologists.   Several have
here placed the seat of sensation and volition.   Rolando
considers it the centre of sensibility, the focus and source
of life.   Fodera supposes it to be the main exciter of
respiration, circulation, digestion and voluntary motion ;
this influence arising mostly from the point where the
pneumogastric nerves arise.   Treviranus believes it the
centre of animal life.   M. Serres considers it the principal seat of sensibility, and M. Flourens regards it as the
source or centre of vitality, and thinks that all other parts
of the nervous system are dependent upon it.   M. Grainger thinks the reason of its great importance is because
the pneumo-gastric, the *excitor* nerve of respiration is attached to it.

Without subscribing to the correctness of these doc-
trines, for we regard this part as subordinate in function
to other portions of the brain, we readily admit that its
office is undoubtedly important, though probably the corpora olivaria or the eminences formed by a dense oblong
nucleus of cineritous matter, from which the pneumo-
gastric nerves arise, are the seat of the most important
functions.

" It is highly probable," says Solly, " that the corpus
olivare is a central point, from whence emanates that peculiar power which the system of respiratory nerves
conduct, and by which they call the respiratory muscles
into action independently of volition.   In support of the
opinion that the respiratory muscles are dependent on

the corpus olivare for their stimulus to contraction, the results of two or three experiments may be related.

"A section of the spinal cord made above the origin of the intercostal nerves simply annihilates, as regards the respiratory movement, the power of the intercostal muscles. A section above the phrenic nerve induces paralysis of the diaphragm ; while a section exactly at the origin of the par vagum, and therefore through the corpus olivare, occasions a total cessation of every respiratory movement and instant death. If the section, however, be made above the corpus olivare, then the whole of the respiratory movements take place as usual. Is it not, then, from this point, and this only, that they draw their power of motion? A section of the par vagum produces no such effect; the section must destroy the corpus olivare before total interruption to the respiratory action can take place."

In respect to the pyramidal bodies, there is a peculiarity deserving of attention. I allude to what is called their *decussation*. At the place where the medulla oblongata joins the spinal marrow, about an inch and a quarter below the pons Varolii, the fibres of the anterior pyramids obliquely decussate, each to the opposite side : the fibres of the right anterior pyramid plunge into the left half of the spinal marrow, while the fibres from the left anterior pyramid pass into the right half of the cord. This is thought to explain what has been noticed since the time of Hippocrates, that disease or injury of one side of the brain almost uniformly produces paralysis of the opposite side.

In some rare instances, the paralysis is on the same side as the cerebral injury. Such cases are recorded by Baglivi, Morgagni and others.* It is difficult to account

---

* M. Bayle, in the Revue Medicale for 1834, has collected a number of such cases from various writers, and he might have added more.

for such exceptions to a very general law. Some suppose that only part of the filaments decussate. In fact,
in some instances, no decussation has been found.

Perhaps it will be ascertained that in cases of paralysis on the same side of the injury, no decussation exists.
At any rate, whenever such cases are witnessed, if opportunity is afforded, the condition of the fibres of the
anterior columns or motory tract, should be examined.

Pathology has taught us something respecting the functions of the medulla oblongata. M. Hall relates in his
lectures, a case from Mr. Kiernan, of a clot of blood
poured out between the cerebellum and the medulla oblongata, which, by pressing on the latter, caused instant
death, by arresting respiration.

A case of abscess in this part is related by Abercrombie.

CASE XXXIV. — " A child, aged 16 months, whom I
saw only a week before his death, had been in a declin-
ing state of health for ten months The beginning of his
bad health was ascribed to a fall, in which he was supposed to have sustained an injury of the back part of the
head or neck. From this time he was often much oppressed, and had been gradually wasting. Three months
before the time when I saw him, he had squinting, and
appeared to lose the power of the right arm and leg.
The squinting went off after some time, but afterwards
recurred occasionally. The use of the arm and leg was
never entirely recovered. These always appeared weaker than the limbs of the other side, and he seldom attempted to raise the arm at all. He had also suffered
occasionally slight convulsive affections. When I saw
him there was no very marked symptom, except considerable emaciation ; the pulse was frequent, and the

bowels very confined. Much dark-colored matter having been evacuated from his bowels, he seemed to be relieved. After some days, there was a remarkable slowness of the pulse, and in the course of the same day he was attacked with violent convulsions. This recurred several times during two days, and then proved fatal. There was no coma ; the eyes continued sensible during the intervals ; and he took notice of objects a very short time before death.

" *Inspection.* — There were several ounces of fluid in the ventricles of the brain. In the substance of the medulla oblongata, where it is crossed by the pons varolii, there was an abscess which appeared to occupy its whole diameter. It had the appearance of a scrofulous abscess, and was contained in a cyst, the inner surface of which was of a yellow color, and had an appearance of ulceration. There was considerable disease in the glands of the mesentery."

In this instance, I apprehend the abscess was above the corpora olivaria. The same author relates the following case of cartilaginous hardening of a portion of the medulla oblongata.

CASE XXXV. — " A child of 14 years ; unable to walk ; articulation very imperfect ; intelligence very deficient ; deglutition very difficult, liquids swallowed often returning by the mouth and nose ; difficult respiration and frequent convulsions ; but was full in flesh ; had been in this state about a year ; died in six months more.

" *Morbid Appearance.* — Corpora olivaria, crus cerebelli, and tubercula mammillaria in a state of cartilaginous hardness ; other parts sound."

The following is an abridgement of an interesting case,

minutely and admirably related by Dr. James Johnson in the Medico Chirurgical Review for July, 1836.

CASE XXXVI. — "A lady, (Mrs. W.) sister of the celebrated Mrs. Siddons, aged 76 years, had been subject to pain in the back of the head, for 20 years or more. She had also had a distressing and buzzing sound in the ears, especially in the left ear ; but, in other respects, she enjoyed general good health. About two years before the date of my present visit, (Monday, first of February, 1836,) I saw Mrs. W. in Great Russell street, and she then only complained of her usual head-aches. She was preparing to entertain a large dinner party, and invited me to join it. I heard no more of this lady till the above date, when I found her in the most deplorable condition. From having been very embonpoint, she was reduced to a state of comparative emaciation. Her countenance exhibited indescribable distress, and she was unable to utter a single word. She made attempts, indeed, to cloathe her ideas in language ; but only produced inarticulate sounds, which I could not understand. Her maid, however, who had lived long with her, could comprehend her meaning tolerably well. Her intellects were in a state of perfect integrity The loss of speech was the least part of the misfortune. The power of deglutition was so nearly destroyed that it was with the greatest difficulty she could swallow a tea-spoonful of thin jelly, some of which was ejected from the mouth. She was literally perishing by hunger and thirst, though not feeling the common sensations of either. She was unable to put out or to move the tongue. This organ appeared to be shrivelled and drawn up into knots. The present symptoms had commenced about four or five months previously, and increased in the most gradual manner, till they had acquired their present state of intensity. She lingered until the 28th of February, without exhibiting paralysis of any other muscles than those of the tongue and pharynx, and without any aberration of the intellectual faculties.

" *Dissection.* — The vessels of the brain and its membranes were extremely vascular, with some serous effusion between the membranes. The skull was remarkably thick. The substance of the brain was particularly firm. Very little fluid in any of the cavities. The origins of the nerves up to the eighth and ninth pairs were examined, but no lesion could be found. On subverting the brain, the pons varolii and medulla oblongata, together with the superior portion of the medulla spinalis, appeared rather wasted, and their substance somewhat softer than the other parts of the brain. The left vertebral artery, from its emergence from the bony canal to its termination, was dilated to nearly the size of the carotid, and thus pressed on the corpus olivare and corpus pyramidale of that side, which appeared smaller than those of the opposite side.* The organs of the left eighth and ninth nerves were consequently pressed upon. The right vertebral artery was remarkably small. On tracing down the eight pair and the œsophagus through the thorax, we came to an aneurismal pouch or dilatation of the descending aorta, the size of a large walnut, over which the nervus vagus of that side was stretched in the form of a C."

It ought here to be mentioned that cases have been published of disease of the medulla oblongata, and even total loss of portions of the medulla spinalis, without occasioning death or perceptible alteration of functions. M. Velpeau has inserted in his *Archives Generales,* a case

---

* The vertebral artery was afterwards found enlarged at its *origin,* and the probability is that it was so in the bony canal.

of disorganization of the medulla oblongata, without disturbance of function.   Such cases contradict all we
know of the functions of these parts.   With M. Bouillaud, I am disposed to believe the narrators of them have
either erred in the observation of symptoms, or in describing the alteration of the parts in question.

We thus learn from pathology and other sources of
knowledge, that although the functions of the medulla
oblongata are not fully understood, that they are very
important, and we may reasonably conclude that disease
of this organ is not a very rare occurrence ; that some
alarming and 'many marvelous and yet mysterious affections, accompanied by difficulty of respiration and deglutition and disturbance of digestion, arise from functional
or organic disease of this part of the system.

MEDULLA SPINALIS.

This is a long cylindrical cord, extending from the medulla oblongata through the vertebral canal ; consisting,
externally, of a layer of medullary substance, and containing within its centre a portion of cineritious matter.
This cord is made up of two halves, placed laterally to
each other, as regards the mesial line of the body.   The
division of these halves is marked by a deep anterior and
a shallow posterior fissure, and each lateral portion has
two fissures, the anterior and posterior lateral.   Thus
each half of the spinal cord is divided into three columns
of longitudinal fibres.

It is generally supposed that the fibres of the anterior
columns transmit the commands of the will, and the posterior convey sensation ; and, by Sir Charles Bell, the

middle column is believed to be connected with respiration. But all this has not been satisfactorily established, though there is not much doubt that the spinal cord consists of distinct tracts of fibres for the transmission of volition and sensation, but that they are separately arranged in the anterior and posterior portions of the cord, has not been proved. As regards the respiratory tract of Sir C. Bell, most physiologists consider his views on this subject incorrect. Dr. Hall, however, regards the respiratory as entirely distinct from the other subdivisions of the nervous system : aud differs from Sir C. Bell, in viewing the respiratory as but *a part* of a more extensive system — as an *excited* and not a *spontaneous* function — as *originating*, when the cerebrum is removed, in the pneumogastric *as its excitor*, and not in the medulla oblongata.

With the lateral portions of the spinal cord are connected the vertebral or spinal nerves. These consist of thirty-one pairs joined to the cord by two setts of filaments, called the anterior and posterior roots.

The anterior roots are smaller than the posterior, and have been proved by Sir C. Bell and others, to be the instruments of volition — the conductors of the will from the brain to the voluntary muscles. The posterior roots are not only larger than the anterior, but are distinguished by passing through a distinct ganglion near their connection with the spinal cord. These convey sensation through the medium of the cord to the brain, the seat of consciousness.

The cineritious matter of the cord is disposed in two crescentic portions, one in each half of the cord, the concavity of each looking outward, and the two portions connected by a band of grey matter. This grey matter extends through the cord, and is continuous with that in the medulla oblongata, the pons varolii, the optic thalami, and the straited bodies.

The fibrous or medullary portion of the cord envelopes the grey matter, and on approaching the medulla oblongata, the anterior fibres cross and extend to the convolutions of the cerebrum, and the lamina of the cerebellum. The mode of attachment of the spinal nerves to the cord, does not seem to be well ascertained. Some authorities conclude that they are connected with the grey, and others with the medullary, portion of the cord.

Mr. Grainger[*] has recently examined with care the connection of the two roots of the spinal nerves with the cord, and says, " after the two roots have perforated the theca vertebralis, and so reached the surface of the cord, their fibres begin to separate from each other ; of the fibres, some are lost in the white substance, whilst others, entering more deeply into the lateral furrows, are found to continue their course, nearly in a right angle with the spinal cord itself, as far as the grey substance in which they are lost ; " and he adds, " From numerous examinations, I am induced to believe, that whenever the white fibres of the nervous system become connected with the grey substance, whether in the different masses of the brain, in the spinal cord, or in the ganglions, the arrangement is similar to what is seen in the section of the corpus striatum. The fibres become, as it were, encrusted with the grey matter, a disposition which may be seen by a careful inspection in the convolutions of the cerebrum, in which the radiating fibres of the crus cerebri are observed like delicate striæ."

----

[*] Observations on the Structure and Functions of the Spinal Cord. By R. D. Grainger, Lecturer on Anatomy and Physiology. London, 1837.

He further states that the cerebral nerves are likewise attached both to the grey and to the fibrous substance.

From such anatomical facts and observations we are enabled to see the connections of the spinal cord and its nerves with the various parts of the brain and cerebellum. We also now understand, as has been already stated, why disease of one hemisphere of the brain produces paralysis of the opposite side of the body, owing to the decussation of the anterior fibres of the medulla oblongata. That this effect results from the decussation, is rendered quite certain, from the fact that injuries of one side of the brain above the medulla oblongata, affect the opposite side, while injuries of the spinal cord below the medulla oblongata affect the same side. Sir A. Cooper divided, in a dog, the right half of the spinal cord at the interval between the occiput and atlas, which produced paralysis of the injured side.

Some of the most important functions of the spinal column may now be readily inferred. Such as diseases of it producing paralysis of the parts below, and that injury confined to the anterior portion, producing loss of voluntary motion, by depriving the will of all command over the muscles below, but not producing loss of sensation, while injury of the posterior column affects sensation, but not voluntary motion.

According to the experiments and investigations of Marshall Hall, the spinal cord is not a mere conductor of nervous power—of volition and sensation, but is a generator of nervous power, totally distinct from sensation and volition, called the reflex power.

This he proved by dividing the spinal cord of a frog, just below the occiput, which caused a cessation of all spontaneous motion, but on pinching the toes, both lower extremities were moved, which motion could not have been produced through the agency of the nerve conveying the mandates of the will, but by exciting a nerve of sensation, which made an impression upon the cord that caused the motion. He believes the spinal cord is not a mere appendage of the brain, but that a portion of it is for the manifestation of this independent power, and that this portion constitutes the true spinal cord. He also goes further, and suggests that " there is a series of incident *excitor nerves*, and of reflex *motor nerves*, which, with the true *spinal* marrow as their centre or axis, constitute the *true* spinal system, as distinguished from the *cerebral*, through which the muscular action is excited ; and that the *ingestion* and *egestion* of air and food, and the action of the *orifices* and *sphincters* of the body are dependent upon this system."

It would thus seem, that the spinal nerves are composed of four, instead of two, classes of nerves, and transmit different impressions. That two are connected with the brain, and, as has been observed, are for the transmission of sensation and volition, and of the two others connected with the cord, one transmits impressions to the grey matter of the cord, and excites its particular and independent powers, while the other transmits to the muscles the effects of the powers thus excited. These nerves, passing from the skin, &c. to the true spinal cord, Dr. H. calls the *incident nerves*, and those that proceed from the true spinal cord to the muscles, the *reflex nerves*. It should, however, be borne in mind, that these different nerves have not been demonstrated.

These views of Dr. Hall are by many deemed quite fanciful, and as not adding any thing of importance to our knowledge of the nervous system ; but in my opinion they are deserving of attention and further examination. They certainly explain some of the phenomena of spasmodic and convulsive diseases, heretofore very mysterious. It should, however, be recollected, that a new language is employed, new terms, as incident and reflex, are used, and may give the appearance of new discovery to much that was known before. I should also say, that similar views were advanced a long time since by Prochaska, and more recently by Mayo, but by neither were evolved into a system.

But let us resort to pathology to learn further respecting the functions of the spinal cord. From pathology we learn that the division of the spinal marrow or severe laceration or pressure of it produces immediate and complete paralysis, but if the injury be partial, then only certain muscles will be paralysed. Instances of this kind are so numerous, and are so frequently occurring, that it is not necessary to cite the particulars of cases.*

We learn from pathology that disease of the anterior portion of the spiral cord, produces loss of motion only.

The following is a case of this kind from *Ollivier on Diseases of the Spinal Marrow.*

CASE XXXVII. — Louis Spreval, a fusileer in the 5th demi-brigade of Veterans, entered the Maison Royale de Charenton, on the 17th October, 1806. No precise information could be collected respecting his complaints anterior to this period. During the first seven or eight

---

* There are said to be some extraordinary exceptions. Cases have been collected by Magendie, Velpeau, and others, of disorganization and division of the spinal cord, that did not deprive the parts below of sensation and motion. Velpeau explains this by supposing that a communication of nervous influence may be kept up between the upper and lower portions by means of the lateral branches. I have before referred to these cases, and expressed my opinion of them in the words of M. Bouillaud, " that it is probable the observers committed some error either in observing symptoms or in describing the alterations of the spinal cord."

years of his residence there, he was taciturn, indolent, idle. It was difficult to get him from his bed. Few rational answers could be obtained from him on any subject. His gait was unsteady, and his lower extremities tottered as he walked. The motions of his arms were free, pulse slow and feeble, appetite, digestion, and sleep natural. Sometimes he had transient paroxysms of maniacal excitement. By the end of nine years, his lower extremities had become completely paralytic, *yet they preserved their sensibility.* For many years his urine and stools came away involuntarily his intellectual faculties became quite abolished, he merely ate, drank, and slept. At length, he died, on the 2d March, 1823, in consequence of a bowel complaint.

Dissection. — Marasmus. Cranium like ivory, and thrice the natural thickness. Dura mater thickened. Arachnoid healthy, as was, also, the pia mater, except where it covers the pons varolii and corpora olivaria, where it was thickened, condensed, and of a blueish color. On raising the pia mater from the corpora olivaria and pyramidalia, these bodies were found softened and converted into a sort of fluid pulp, which condition obtained along the whole point of the spinal marrow downwards, while it could be traced upwards to the thalami nervorum opticorum, corpora striata and even into some of the convolutions of the brain. All other parts of the brain were sound in appearance, as was the cerebellum, excepting the commissures of the latter, which was indurated, forming a striking contrast with the neighboring softened parts. The *anterior roots* of the spinal nerves had lost their natural consistence ; while the *posterior* part of the medulla spinalis, and the *nerves* which issue from it, were perfectly sound. It is rare, as our author observes, to find such an exact correspondence between the symptoms during life and the appearances after death.

This case is certainly we think, decisive of the difference of the functions of the anterior and posterior spinal roots.

Case XXXVIII. — In the Annales de Chimie et de Physique, Magendie notices the case of a man who had lost the use of his arms, but retained completely their sensibility, and in whose body it was found, that the posterior roots of the nerves, which form the axillary plexus, were entire, while their anterior roots were reduced by the loss of medullary matter almost to their mere membranous covering. (Vol. xxiii, 432.) In the same paper *another* case, to the same effect is mentioned on the authority of Royer Collard. This person had lost the power of motion over the whole body, but preserved sensibility ; and on examining the body after death, R. C. found evident disease in the whole anterior part of the spinal cord. (435.) The last we shall notice is described with great minuteness and apparent fidelity by Dr. Koreff, in the 4th vol. of Magendie's Journal. There existed complete palsy of both legs, and imperfect palsy of both arms, while the sensibility was every where preternaturally acute. " The medullary matter of the cord was singularly contracted in volume, the anterior part of the upper half was reddish colored, and, as it were, macerated, the roots of the nerves inserted there, were so wasted as to be hardly discernible, but the posterior roots were unnaturally large."

Usually injury of one side of the spinal column produces paralysis of the same side, but there are some few cases recorded where the paralysis was on the side opposite to the disease of the cord. The following is an instance.

Case XXXIX. — A woman had experienced, for many years, smart convulsive twitchings of the left lower

13

extremity at each menstrual period. At 40 years of age the catamenia ceased, and then the member above mentioned became completely paralytic. Sometime afterwards, convulsive twitchings were felt in the left arm, and the woman died comatose. On inspecting the body and opening the spine, the arachnoid and pia mater covering the spinal marrow, were found inflamed opposite to the last dorsal, and first lumbar vertebræ. The spinal marrow itself was reddened and softened on its right side, but perfectly sound in appearance on the *left.*— *Portal Anat. Med. tom.* iv. *p.* 116.

Sometimes after entire loss of sensation and voluntary motion from disease or injury of the spinal cord, the limbs thus paralysed, contract on irritating the nerves of the extremities. Mr. Mayo alludes to this, and Mr. Grainger relates the following case as pathological evidence in support of the reflex theory of Dr. Hall.

Case XL. — A girl about fifteen years of age, who was a patient of Mr. Crosse at the Norfolk and Norwich hospital a few years since, was affected with angular curvature of the spine, producing insensibility and paralysis of the lower extremities. On tickling *the soles of her feet,* which, as an experiment was often done, the legs were immediately slightly retracted, although the patient said she felt nothing ; it was further remarked, that on touching the *other parts of the feet or the legs* in the same manner, no effect was produced. But such effects are not always observed after injuries of the cord that destroy sensation and volition.

In the New York Alms House, I saw a female patient who had been confined there nearly a year, with complete insensibility and paralysis of the lower extremities, in consequence of an injury of the lumbar vertebræ. I have repeatedly tried, since reading the case just quoted, to produce some motion of the limbs by irritating the nerves of the feet, but have not been able to produce the least motion. Instances of like failure were recently adduced by Mr. Brereton, and Dr. Whiting, at a meeting of the Physical Society of Guy's Hospital.*

Inflammation of the spinal cord or its membranes, is generally connected with disease of the brain, so that it is often difficult to say what symptoms are to be attributed to the disease of the cord. It has, however, been found separately inflamed in Tetanus, Hydrophobia, and in Trismus infantum.

Olivier says two symptoms may be considered pathognomonic signs of acute inflammation of the membranes of the spinal cord. One is pain in the dorsal regions, the other general contraction of the muscles of the posterior part of the trunk. It appears, however, from cases published by several authors, that this pain is felt only when the posterior portion of the spinal column is affected with inflammation, but is not manifested when the anterior portion is only inflammed.

Whoever peruses the numerous cases of affections of the spinal cord, published of late, will find that disease of this part of the nervous system may produce functional derangements in most of the organs of the body.

" When we review," says Abercrombie, " the phenomena which have been observed to accompany the diseases of the spinal cord, we find affections of all the principal organs of the body. In the parts connected with the head and neck, we find distortion of the eyes, difficulty and loss of speech, loss of voice, contraction of the jaw, resembling trismus, and difficulty of swallowing, which is said in some cases, to have nearly resem-

---

* London Medical Gazette, April, 1838.

bled hydrophobia. In the viscera of the thorax, there
have been observed oppression, palpitation, and strong
and irregular action of the heart, painful sense of stric-
ture in the region of the diaphragm, and difficulty of
breathing, which, in some cases, has been permanent, and
in others has occurred in paroxysms, resembling asthma.
In the organs of the abdomen and pelvis, we find vomiting, pain of the bowels, resembling colic; tenesmus, involuntary discharge of feces, and retention or incontinence of urine. In the muscular parts, we observe convulsions and paralysis; the convulsions in some cases resembling chorea, in others, tetanus. We are by no means
prepared to say, in the present state of our knowledge,
that all these proceed directly from the affections of the
spinal cord, especially as we observe remarkable diver-
sities and considerable want of uniformity in the symptoms. But the subject presents to us a field of observation which promises most important and most interesting
results."

Several writers have of late attributed various affections to irritation of the spinal cord and the roots of the
spinal nerves. Mr. Tate, in a *Treatise on Hysteria* — a
disease which he thinks is caused by irregular and defective menstruation, says, that in most cases of this disease, spinal tenderness may be detected by pressure on
the vertebræ, and that to this spinal affection is to be attributed the various and fantastic forms that Hysteria
puts on. Mr. Teale* supposes that many neuralgic diseases arise from irritation of the spinal marrow, and relates several cases in support of this opinion. He generally found tenderness over some of the vertebræ in
cases of Neuralgia, and leeching and blistering this part

*A Treatise on Neuralgic Diseases, by Thomas Pridgeu Teale.

cured the disease. But it should be noted that no examinations after death are adduced in support of these
opinions, and that all the cases related by Mr. T. occurred but a short time before his work was published,
most of them the same year or year preceding. Too
little time was allowed to test the efficacy of his remedies, as the intermittent character of such diseases is
well known, and that they will appear to yield for a short
time to almost any new remedy. I am aware that this
spinal tenderness may be found in many neuralgic and
hysterical disorders, though I am inclined to consider it
rather the result of a general increase of sensibility, than
a disease of any one part of the nervous system. One
thing deserving of notice in injuries of the spinal marrow, and the same is true of injuries of nerves, which
cause an interruption of nervous influence, is, the tendency of some of the parts thus cut off, to inflame, to
mortify and slough. The mucous membrane lining the
bladder, almost always inflames after an injury of the
spine, and sloughs soon form in various parts, particularly
on those where pressure is made.

To these effects of diminished nervous influence, I shall
recur in another part of this work.

SECTION IV.

FUNCTIONS AND DISEASES OF THE CEREBRAL NERVES.

First Pair. — *Olfactory.* — This pair of nerves appears to be quite differently connected with the brain,
from any of the other cerebral nerves. All the others
are connected with the brain at or near the medulla ob-

13*

longata, but the olfactory, which are solely for the sense
of smell, and are expanded on the lining membrane of
the nose, pass from this membrane through the cribiform
plate of the æthmoid bone, and terminate in the olfactory ganglia in the cribiform fossæ. From these ganglia, commissures, sometimes considered nerves, pass
backwards and divide into three portions, two of which
are attached to the cineriteous substance at the posterior
part of the anterior lobes of the cerebrum, and one to
the anterior part of the middle lobe.

Some persons are destitute of the sense of smell from
birth, and this defect is hereditary, though the organic
cause is not always known. Blows on the head sometimes abolish it. Conolly tells of a man who lost the
sense of smell in consequence of an injury behind the
ears. Ulceration and disease affecting the pituitary membrane, sometimes destroys it. According to Magendie,
affections of the nasal branch of the fifth pair of nerves,
which branch is a nerve of general sensation, abolish the
sense of smell. The loss of this sense is a symptom occurring in some nervous diseases, as hysteria and epilepsy.

The nerves themselves have been found diseased.
Foville says he often found the olfactory nerves in the
insane, hard and transparent. In some instances, the
sense of smell is destroyed on one side only. Mr. Swan*
relates the case of a man who complained of an extremely violent pain in the right side of the forehead by
the crista galli, with entire loss of smell in the right
nostril, the left not being affected. He was relieved from
pain, and the sense of smell restored, by bleeding, ca-
thartics and low regimen. In this case there was proba-

---

* A Dissertation on the Treatment of Morbid Local Affections of
the nerves. By Joseph Swan, London.

bly inflammation of the right olfactory ganglion in the cribiform fossæ.

Sometimes, exposure to strong or very disagreeable odors destroys the sense of smell. The following is related by Dr. Graves, in the *Medical Gazette*, for 1834.

CASE XLI. — " I had lately an opportunity of observing a very singular case of the total loss of the sense of smelling, occasioned by exposure to the effects of a very strong and disagreeable odor. Mr. ——, formerly a captain in a yeomanry corps, was attended by Mr. Barker, of Britain-street, and myself. He was affected with ascites, and in the course of conversation one day, mentioned that in the Irish rebellion of 1798, information was received by the magistrates, that five hundred pikes were concealed in one of the markets in this city, buried at the bottom of a large cess-pool, which was filled with the offscourings of the market, and all manner of filth. He proceeded to the place, and superintended the work of emptying out the cess-pool, at the bottom of which the concealed arms were found as specified. During this operation, he was exposed to most abominable effluvia, and suffered greatly at the time from the stench. Next day, he found that he had become entirely insensible to odors, and since that, now a period of thirty-six years, he has remained completely deprived of the sense of smelling. From this, it appears, that, as exposure to very intense light may produce amaurosis, so exposure to intense odors may produce a corresponding affection of the olfactory nerve."

Second Pair. — Optic Nerves. — From their expansion in the retina, they pass through the coats of the eye, through the skull at the foramen opticum of the sphenoid bone, and on the processus olivarius of this bone, they appear to unite, but soon separate, spreading laterally, and sending a few fibres to the tuber cinereum, take a course over the crus cerebri, each nerve dividing into an external and internal branch. The external branch is lost in the external geniculate body; the internal goes to the optic tubercles or Quadrigminal bodies, which are considered the appropriate ganglia of the optic nerves. Mr. Solly says they divide, after passing the crura cerebri, into superficial and deep, and that the former is the one described by Anatomists, and that the latter goes *into* the substance of the thalamus and corpus geniculatum, its fibres being separated by neurine, and lost in the substance of the thalamus.

Whether the optic nerves unite or decussate, is not fully ascertained. In fishes, whose eyes are so placed that light from one object cannot impinge on both, they completely cross, and have a membrane between them. Mr. Mayo supposes the arrangement is such that the outer and the inner side of each opposite retina is formed by one and the same nerve, and thus it is that a single impression is conveyed to the sensorium, though each retina receives the impression.

According to M. Ozanam, of Lyons, who has zealously investigated the structure of the optic nerves, they do not decussate, but are separated from each other by a thin membrane, filled with medullary substance. M. Ozanam placed between two plates of glass, in a solar microscope, the optic nerves of a person who had just died of encephalitis; the nerves were detached three lines before their juncture, and six lines beyond this point. The image thus formed was so magnified, as to appear six feet long, and three feet broad, thus occupying an area of eighteen square feet; each nerve seemed to be eight inches round, and the membrane or interposed pouch, two feet across. This pouch seemed filled with medullary matter, the consistence of cream. From this account it appears that the optic nerves do not decussate, but may communicate by means of the medullary matter in the pouch alluded to.*

The optic nerves are frequently diseased, producing partial or complete blindness, though the same calamity may arise from disease of the brain or of the eye itself, from tumors pressing on the nerves, and even from injury or disease of branches of the fifth pair of nerves. Thus, M. Demours relates that amaurosis followed the extirpation of a cyst, situated three inches above the left eyebrow, the day after the operation.

In amaurosis, the optic nerves have been found atrophied and shrunk to one third their natural size. Foville found them hard and partially transparent in a lunatic who had long been tormented with horrible images. In the Connecticut Retreat for the Insane, was a patient thus tormented, and who appeared to have no mental aberration but what was connected with this derangement of vision — or the sight of horrible beings approaching him. His eyes were considerably red, and pressure on the eye ball gave great pain. I apprehend that in this case there was some disease of the optic nerve, though there was undoubtedly, at least a part of the time, disease of the brain. Sometimes he saw and would describe the beings that tormented him, and appear to realize that they were but phantoms created by his disordered nerves, and at such times would give but little attention to them, but at others he believed in their reality, and acted accordingly.

I have found the optic nerves unnaturally hard, and the membranes covering them at their union very

---

* Archives Generales, 1832.

highly injected with blood and thickened, in four individuals who died of delirium tremens, and who, for some time previous to death were terrified by images of the most vile and horrid animals.

In the 24th volume of the Medico Chirurgical Review, is an interesting case related by the editor, Dr. James Johnson, of a man who died of apoplexy, but who had long been tormented with a series of the most dazzling images by day and night. Sometimes they assumed the form of angels with flaming swords. The intellectual powers were not disturbed. On dissection, an hydated mass was found pressing upon the optic nerves, which were reduced to the size of threads, and of a soft consistence.

Functional disorders of the optic nerves are quite common, producing often the most bizarre hallucinations. I have a patient who occasionally is not able to see but one half of an object. This appears to arise from pressure of blood in the head, as it is accompanied by pain of the forehead, and relieved by bleeding.

Demours relates that Madame de Pompadour took cold in the Park of Versailles, in 1762, and awoke the next day, incapable of seeing but the half of any object she looked at with the left eye. She could only see on looking at the face of a person near her the right cheek and corresponding side of the nose. Only half of the iris was capable of dilation and contraction. The complaint disappeared in about two months.

Mr. Abernethy, the celebrated surgeon, was subject, it seems, to such attacks. " On one occasion," he observes, " when I was riding, my horse's head and my own came pretty near together. On putting the spurs to him, and pulling the bridle, he threw up his head and struck me with it right on the nose. The blood flowed from it, just as if it had been streaming from an arm after you had introduced the lancet. I got off, went into a stable near at hand, washed my face, and squeezed the bones into their proper situation as well as I could. The people were certainly very kind, and wished to send for a surgeon to me; but I told them I would rather they sent for a hackney coach, which they did, and I went home in it. I then perceived, for the first time in my life, an imperfection in my sight. I could not see more than two-thirds of an object. First of all, however, I should tell you, my vision was indistinct, but I found it arose from the eclipse of the *third* of every object on the right hand. I ascertained this particular as I went home, because if I saw such a long name as my own, for instance, *A-ber-ne-thy*, in a bookseller's shop window, or any such place, I could see *A-ber-knee*, but I could not see the *thigh* at all. Well, I looked with one eye, then I looked with the other, and I looked with both, but still I perceived that the third of every object was eclipsed, on what I may call my right side.. Now this sort of case is alluded to by Dr. Wollaston, and he contends that it might be a defect in the optic nerve. Well, I was telling all this to a medical friend of mine — a very clever man, and he said it was impossible. I said, ' Well, I do not know whether it is impossible or not, but I know that what I tell you is true.' It afterwards happened that he had a fall from his horse, I believe, or something of that kind, and he had the same imperfection of sight, the eclipse of the objects being on the opposite side. I said to him, there was only one thing I regretted, which was, that when I was in that state, I had not squinted, to have seen how the things would have looked then. He told me he was convinced it arose from the nerve. But I said, ' did you squint?' ' No,' said he, ' I never thought of squinting.' But since that time I have been entertained with it often, and often without having had any blow;

and I have, on those occasions, squinted too, and it is just the same. And let those who can account for it as arising from a decussation of the nerve, do it; my own opinion is, that it arises from the irregular actions of the retina. You know there are people who see ghosts, and goblins, and so on; they absolutely see men and women; you know all that, I dare say."*

Symptoms very similar result from wounds of the brain and optic nerves, as the following case from Larrey exhibits.

CASE XLII. — Læcour, a soldier in the Royal Guard, received, 19th November, 1820, a thrust of a sharp foil between the globe of the right eye, (which was not touched,) and the internal parietes of the orbit, the weapon penetrating, by all accounts, three inches or thereabouts. The wound healed, but Læcour, when looking with the right eye alone, could only see the perpendicular half of objects placed in the antero-posterior axis of that eye. As it was with that half of the eye next to the nose, which Læcour saw objects, so when these objects were carried towards the left of the patient, he lost sight of them, *in toto*, at a time when they could be distinctly seen with the left eye, if open. Thus it appeared, that the inner or nasal half of the retina was paralytic. In this state he was seen by the members of the *Faculte de Medicine*, three months after the accident occurred. A few weeks subsequently, Læcour committed some excess, was seized with phrenitis and enteritis at the same time, and died on the fourth day of the disease.

---

* Lectures on Anatomy, Surgery and Pathology, by John Abernethy F. R. S., vol. 1.

Necrologic Examination. — Invaginations of the small intestines and peritoneal inflammation were observed in the abdomen, but the head was the greatest object of research, on account of the retinal paralysis before described. It was found that the point of the foil had pierced the orbital plate, and grooved the under surface of the anterior lobe of the right hemisphere, passing obliquely behind the point of the falx, and above the decussation of the optic nerves, stopping under the inferior paries of the left lateral ventricle. This tract was marked by a kind of reddish clot of fibrinous substance, but without any appearance of suppuration. Immediately surrounding this clot, the cerebral substance was yellow, and manifestly altered in consistence to about half a line in depth. Some slight serosity was effused under the left hemisphere.

Third Pair : — Oculo Muscular. — Arises from the inner side of crus cerebri, where it dips beneath the annular tubercle, and divides; one portion of it is connected with the black matter of the crus, the other with the motor tract of the cord. It is purely a voluntary nerve of the eye, perfectly under the control of the will, and goes to the levator muscle of the eye and eye lid, to the depressor muscle of the eye, to the rectus internus, and to the inferior oblique, and the lenticular ganglion.

Affections of this nerve lead to Ptosis or paralysis of the upper eye lid. The following is a case illustrative of this. It is described in a letter to Sir C. Bell, and published in his " *Appendix to the Papers on the Nerves.*"

Nov. 24, 1825.

CASE XLIII. — " The master of a small trading vessel applied for advice. The most prominent and obvious symptom of the case was *Ptosis*, or paralysis of the up-

14

per eyelid. Suspecting that there might be a general
affection of the third nerve, or motor nerve, I desired
him to look to the ground ; he attempted it, but was ut-
terly unable to accomplish his intention. He was also
told to look upwards, and then inwards ; in both which
he failed.

"He could close and wink with the eyelids when we
touched the cilia, proving that the *portio dura*, and the
branches of the fifth, possessed of their sensibility and
power.

"Now, forcibly separating the eyelids, and desiring
him to close them, while I still held them open, I could
distinctly see the eyeball turn upwards, which I supposed
to indicate that the fourth nerve still influenced the troch-
learis muscle.

"He had the power of looking outwards, accomplished by the sixth, which was not included in the paralytic
affection. He saw well, save that the fallen lid interfered with vision. He had been troubled with this affection nearly a fortnight, attended with slight head-ache,
and some symptoms of derangement of the stomach and
bowels.   SAMUEL JOHN STRATFORD."

Referring to the observations of the ingenious writer
of the letter, Sir C. Bell remarks, "they are important,
since the defect is proved to be in a cerebral nerve, and
therefore to imply an affection of the brain, and to threat-
en apoplexy."

Fourth Pair ; — Inner Oculo Muscular or Pathetic. —
This is the smallest of the cerebral nerves, and arises
from the intercerebral commissure or from that portion of
the process extending from the cerebellum to the testis
to which the valve of Vieussens is attached. Its distribution is to the superior oblique muscle of the eye. This
nerve and its functions are thus commented on by Sir

C. Bell, in his " *Exposition of the Natural System of the Nerves.*"

" This is a fine nerve, which takes its origin from the brain, at a part remote from all the other nerves which run into the orbit. It threads the intricacies of the other nerves without touching them, and is entirely given to one muscle, the superior oblique. We may observe, too, that this singularity prevails in all animals.

"If it be asked now, as it has been asked for some hundred years past, why the fourth nerve goes into the orbit, where there are so many nerves, why it is so distant in its origin from the other nerves, and why it sends off no twig or branch, but goes entirely to one muscle of the eye? the answer is, to provide for the insensible and instinctive rolling of the eyeball; and to associate this motion of the eyeball with the winking motions of the eyelids; to establish a relation between the eye and the extended respiratory system; all tending to the security or preservation of the organ itself."

Fifth Pair : — Trigeminal. — This is one of the most important nerves of the body, and one that requires much study in order to understand all the symptoms produced by affections of its various branches. It is, says Sir C. Bell, the universal nerve of sensation to the head and face, to the skin, the surface of the eye, the cavities of the nose, the mouth, the tongue. It has a double origin, a ganglion at its root, and therefore has a double function, sensation and motion. Mr. Bell regards it as the first of the spinal nerves.

The connection of the roots of this nerve with the brain is different. The motor tract arises from the inter-cerebral commissure, very close to the cerebellum; running from this origin concealed by the fibres of the pons Varolii, it emerges through the fibres of this body near the crura cerebelli, close to the spot where the sensory division passes through and then becomes connected with this portion.

The sensory tract appears to be connected with the posterior columns of the spinal cord about an inch and a half below the pons Varolii, and ascends through the fibres of that body at the point where the motory tract emerges. In connection with the motory tract it enters the process of the dura mater extending from the clinoid process of the sphenoid bone to the fibrous portion of the temporal, and beneath the anterior part of this membrane, in the tempora-sphenoidal fossa, the sensory or posterior tract forms or enters into the semilunar or Gasserion ganglion of the *fifth nerve*. It emerges from the ganglion in three divisions, the opthalmic, the superior maxillary and the inferior maxillary. The opthalmic is the smallest and enters the orbit at the superior lacerated foramen of the sphenoid bone. The superior maxillary is larger and passes through the foramen rotundum, and the inferior maxillary, which is the largest, passes through the foramen ovale.

The sensory portion of the fifth pair is distributed by numerous branches and filaments on the surface of the mucous membrane of the nose, of the palate, the pulpy structure of the teeth in both jaws, the papilla of the tongue, and the many parts connected with the orbit, the lachrymal apparatus, the conjunctiva, and the skin covering the face.

The motory tract or anterior portion of the fifth pair, is smaller than the posterior and does not enter the semilunar ganglion, but passes behind or on its inner side, connected to it by membranes, and goes out at the foramen ovale with the third branch of the sensory tract and is distributed to the muscles concerned in the motions of mastication, the temporal, masseter, pterygoid and buccinnator. Such is the connection of this nerve with the brain, as described by Solly, and as I have myself traced it, but the pursuit of this connection is intricate and difficult, as any one who undertakes to make out the exact point of connection, will find. It is therefore not surprising that others should assign different points of connection. Hence some say that the motor branch arises from the fibrous bundles of the pyramidal bodies, and the sensory from the interior of the restiform bodies.

From numerous experiments of Fodera, Magendie, Bell, Mayo and others, performed on animals by dividing different branches of the fifth pair of nerves, it appears to be well established that all the branches from that portion of the fifth that enters the semilunar ganglion, the posterior, are nerves of sensation only, and that those of the other division, the anterior, are nerves of motion.

I need not recapitulate the numerous experiments that establishes these facts.

One division of the fifth nerve deserves, however, separate consideration. It is the Gustatory nerve, the most important portion of the inferior maxillary nerve. By experiments on the branches of this nerve, it seems they confer sensibility on the tongue and also the sense of taste ; that division of them does not effect the motion of the tongue, but destroys its sensibility and the power of taste.

Subsequent experiments tend however to show that this division destroys the sense of taste only at the tip of the tongue.

Still later researches serve to show that several nerves probably contribute to the perfection of the sense of taste, that the gustatory nerve is most essential; that it is distributed to the end of the tongue, where that sense is most perfect ; but that the lingual (hyo glossal) though a nerve of motion, as it goes to the muscles of the tongue.

14*

is essential to tasting, and the glosso-pharyngeal supplies the mucous membrane of the base of the tongue and the muscles of the pharynx and confers special sensibility on these parts, which contribute to the perfection of the sense of taste.

Thus it seems from what we at present know that taste is a composite sense, made up of impressions on the nerves of touch and the proper nerves of taste and even those of smell.

Some suppose that Meckel's Ganglion — the Spheno Palatine ganglion plays an important part and connects the senses of smell, taste, hearing and sight.

Some singular cases have been published of facial paralysis in which the common sensation of one half the tongue was annihilated, while the sense of taste was unimpaired ; and others in which the common sensibility of the left half of the tongue was but little impaired, while the sense of taste was lost.

Pathology has thrown some light on the functions of the fifth pair of nerves. The following is an interesting case of disease of certain branches of this nerve.

CASE XLIV. — " M. Serres has lately observed a very curious case at the hospital of La Pitie. An epileptic patient had, six months since, an inflammation of the right eye, with closure of the pupil, and a very dense opacity of the transparent cornea. The loss of sight on that side was necessarily the result.

In the early part of the month of August, it was discovered that the *conjunctiva* was so insensible, that you might pass between the eyelids and the globe of the eye the fibrils of a feather without the patient's perceiving it. The right nostril was deeply insensible to the introduction of a foreign body. The sulphate of quinine put on the right side of the tongue was not tasted. The gums on the same side were soft, fungous, blackish, and detached from the bones. The teeth were almost all carious; many of them had fallen out. The gums on the opposite side were also diseased, but less so than on the right. Lastly the hearing was very indistinct on the right side. The patient at length died of a chronic affection of the brain, which had disorganised a large part of that viscus, without producing any remarkable phenomena. The inspection of the body was made in the presence of M. M. Serres, Magendie, Lisfranc, Georget, and many other distinguished men. They at first read the details of the case, which we have summarily given.

The fifth pair of nerves on the right side presented a very remarkable alteration. At its origin it was soft, yellowish and almost gelatinous. This appearance extended a line or two in depth towards the *tuber annulare*. The nerve might now be traced toward it without offering any change either in color or consistency. The nerve was torn in attempting to turn out the brain. The back part of the nerve, as it passes on the petrous portion, had the same appearance, it was soft and yellowish, excepting, however, the filaments which were perfectly healthy. On the petrous portion, before the plexus, the nervous filaments were separated by an infiltration of serum, but they had preserved their firmness. The ganglion was yellow, and had a projection not observed on the opposite side. By measuring on the petrous portion, the size of the nerves of each side, it was found that the one on the left side, which was healthy, was four lines and a half, and the other only three lines. The anterior chamber of the eye had disappeared, by the adhesion of the cornea to the iris.

The coincidence of a *lesion of one of the nerves of the fifth pair*, with the alteration of the *structure* of the *eye* and the *gums*, with the *loss* of the senses of *hearing* and *taste*, is particularly interesting, as it confirms the result obtained by M. Magendie, when he divided the nerves of the fifth pair.

One circumstance that ought not to be forgotten, is, that in this patient the muscular filaments of the affected nerve were healthy, and that mastication was not impeded. It is the intention of M. Serres to publish this case more in detail."*

Sixth Pair : — Abducentes. — This nerve is generally said to arise from the motor . tract just below the pons Varolii, or from the pyramidal bodies, but according to Mr. Grainger, whom I think correct, a part of this nerve may be traced deep into the medulla oblongata, until it reaches the grey matter.

It directs its course forward and penetrates the dura mater, half an inch below the posterior clinoid process, crosses the carotid artery, and here is joined by some filaments from the sympathetic nerve, which accompanies it into the orbit. It is distributed to the abductor (rectus externus) muscle of the eye. Prof. Pannizza, of Pavia, has shown, however, that this branch of the sympathetic does not communicate with the sixth, as is generally supposed, but is merely entwined around it. The sixth appears to be merely a voluntary nerve of the eye, and physiologically but a part of the third. If affected, strabismus results. Pressure upon it causes this, as is seen by Case XXVIII, already quoted.†

Seventh Pair : — Facial, or Portio Dura. — Arises from the lateral part of the medulla oblongata, just below the pons Varolii, in the groove between this and the pyramidal body. It passes forward to the internal au-

---

* Lancet, vol. vii.   † See Appendix A.

ditory foramen, and into the aqueduct of Fallopius, and quits the skull at the inferior orifice of this canal, called the stylo-mastoid foramen, between the styloid and mastoid process, just below the ear. It gives some branches to the muscles attached to the styloid process of the temporal bone, and passing through the parotid gland, is distributed to the platysma myoides, and the muscles of the face. It is a nerve of motion solely, and conveys no sensibility. Diseases and paralytic affections of this nerve are not uncommon, but since the discoveries of Sir C. Bell, they are understood and generally remedied. The following is not an uncommon case. Mr. ——, a young man, applied to me, in great terror, for a paralytic affection of one side of his face. It came on suddenly, though he had taken cold, and complained of pain of the ear. General bleeding and mercurial purgatives, and antimonials, soon relieved him. Similar cases are to be found in the medical periodicals of late years.

The following, by Dr. Delafield, of New York, is from the New York Med. and Phys. Journal, for Dec. 1824.

CASE XLV. — " On the 10th of May last, I was requested to see Mrs. Mary Ann Ray. Three weeks before I saw her, she was attacked with violent pain in the head and neck, accompanied with severe inflammatory fever. She was bled, and took a purgative, which relieved the febrile symptoms, but the pain in the head continued, varying in violence, with little abatement, for a fortnight. At this time it became fixed in the right ear, and behind the angle of the jaw ; it subsided, however, in a few days ; and suddenly all the symptoms of partial paralysis of the right side of the face appeared ; and in this case to a greater degree than I had yet seen them. The mouth and tongue were so much affected, that she could articulate very indistinctly, and certain words she could not pronounce at all. The eye was widely open, slightly inflamed, and watering profusely, and by the strongest effort it was not possible to close it. In this situation she had been about a week, gradually growing worse. I ordered six leeches to be placed over the trunk of the portio dura, and a blister to be afterwards applied. She was also directed to take gr. ij. of calomel every other night, and half oz. of sulph. magnes. on the following morning. In a few hours after the application of the leeches, she was much better ; the eye could be half closed, and the mouth was less drawn aside in speaking or smiling. On the 25th, the leeching and blistering were repeated. The improvement was now rapid ; and on the 2d June, fifteen days after I first saw the patient, no vestige of the disease could be discovered."

The following account of an important operation by Dr. Warren, of Boston, in which this nerve and the sub-maxillary nerve were divided, should be called to mind as illustrative of the functions of these nerves.

CASE XLVI. — " Mr. S., aged 70, applied to me, with a dreadful painful complaint in the face, and he wished an operation for his relief. It appeared that he had been first affected without any obvious cause, about fourteen years before. His pains were of two kinds ; first, a constant aching pain, which he compared to the worst tooth-ache ; second, a spasmodic affection which occurred many times during the day. When he had the latter kind of attack, the muscles of the face quivered, the face became red and swelled, the eyes were filled with tears, and his intellect was for the moment suspended. For the last four years, he had not been free from pain while awake, and his sleep was short and interrupted

" Respectable practitioners in the part of the country where he lived, had performed three operations, two on the sub-orbitar nerve and its branches, the third on the nerve of the lower jaw, where it comes out on the chin. These operations gave him a degree of relief, but the pain continued with a severity intolerable, and life had become a burden to him.

The pain he described, as beginning near the ear, and thence, darting into the lower and upper jaw, the lips, eye, forehead and scalp. The patient had made himself acquainted with the situation of the nerves of the face, and believed his pain to reside in the facial nerve, which he wished to have divided.

He was informed that an operation such as he wished, might be executed; but that in his case the affection appeared so general, that there was no prospect of a cure; and that, in fact, there were not any cases on record, of a successful division of the facial nerve at its roots, for this disorder. As soon as the patient understood that the operation was practicable, he desired to have it performed, and agreed to enter the Hospital, on account of the superior advantages it afforded over any private situation.

" The operation was thus conducted. An incision, two inches long was carried from the back of the ear downwards in front of the mastoid process. The edge of the parotid gland was then exposed on one side, and on the other, the anterior edge of the mastoid muscles. The dissection being continued between the parotid gland and the mastoid process, the facial nerve was exposed where it crosses this space and passes on the gland, it was divided and a portion cut out. When the nerve was cut, the muscles of the face quivered and were paralysed; but the patient said he merely perceived the division; that it was not attended with an acute pain, and that the principal cause of his sufferings was not reached.

After this operation, it appeared that the pain in the upper part of the face was diminished, perhaps removed.

But the patient now became sensible that the most acute pain, and that which probably had existed first, was seated deeply in the lower jaw, beginning at the zygomatic arch and shooting into the bone. It was entirely independent of the wound made in the operation. From this wound he experienced no inconvenience, was unwilling to speak of it, and scarcely wished it dressed, so greatly was he disappointed at not being relieved from his sufferings. He begged his case might be again taken into consideration, and something more if possible devised for his relief. A meeting of the consulting physicians and surgeons being called, I proposed the operation which is described hereafter, and it being agreed to, was performed nine days after the first.

"An incision was made over the side of the jaw, from the semilunar notch to the inferior edge of the bone. The parotid gland being exposed, was divided as far back as possible, and turned forwards. Then the masseter muscle was divided in the course of its fibres to the bone, and afterwards the edge of the knife being turned forwards, some of the fibres were transversely cut in order to make room over the bone. A trephine, three-quarters of an inch in diameter, was then applied, half an inch below the semilunar notch, midway between the anterior and posterior edges of the jaw; and the circular piece sawed through and removed in two parts, the external table by a lever, the internal by forceps. Between these pieces lay the nerve with its accompanying artery and vein, at the point where they penetrate the bone. At the superior edge of the hole in the bone was seen the large internal maxillary vein, pulsating from the movements of the artery. The submaxillary nerve being now raised on a probe, the patient directly exclaimed that this was the seat of his sufferings. Half an inch of this nerve was cut out, and on examination, it was found to comprehend the branch given to the internal face of the lower jaw. The artery was tied without difficulty. The transverse artery of the face had been previously tied on each side of the wound. A suture was employed to bring together the two parts of the parotid gland, and the wound closed by adhesive plaster.

" The patient said that the pain of this operation could not be compared with that from his disorder. The pain on the wounding and dividing the maxillary nerve was most acute.

" On the evening of the operation, he was relieved from pain, the first time for four years ; and had no return of it afterward. On passing a probe into the wound three or four days after, a branch of nerve in the masseter was touched, and a violent pain produced. The pain did not, however, return, nor had he any threatening of his former attacks. On the nineteenth day from the second operation, his wounds being nearly healed, he left the Hospital perfectly cured of his disease, with the strongest conviction it would not recur, and not a little gratified by his own perseverance."

Eighth Pair : — Auditory or Portio Mollis. — Usually said to arise from the fourth ventricle. Solly says the posterior pyramidal body is its proper ganglion, into which it can be traced. It is connected by cellular membrane to the facial nerve, and enters into the internal auditory canal, and divides into branches which are distributed to the cochlea, the vestibule, and the semicircular canals, and expanded into the pulp that fills the internal ear. This nerve is solely for audition, and its functions are destroyed by disease or pressure on the nerve in its course or origin. Drelincourt relates a case of a tumor between the cerebrum and cerebellum, first causing blind-

15

ness and then deafness. Itard found, in a man who had lost the hearing in the left ear, small tumors lying on the corresponding side of the cerebellum. The auditory nerves have been found atrophied, indurated, and Morgagni says, in one instance, were wanting in cases of deafness.

Loud noises sometimes produce deafness by causing paralysis of the auditory nerve. Usually patients recover their hearing when destroyed from this cause in a few days, but sometimes never. There are no symptoms that indicate with certainty that deafness is owing to the nerve itself being affected. Absence of other causes should lead us to suspect it.*

Ninth Pair: — Glosso Pharyngeal. — This has by some been associated with the Pneumogastric or the tenth pair. It arises from the corpus olivare just above the pneumogastric and goes to the muscles of the Pharynx and tongue. Mr. Bell thinks it essential to complete respiration and some have supposed that branches of it are sent to the papilla of the tongue, and that it contributes to the sense of taste. It is often involved in disease ; it was in the cases already quoted from Dr. Bright, page 124. Its functions are still obscure. Dr. Reid† has performed numerous experiments on animals, to determine the functions of this nerve and his conclusions are as follows.

" From a full review of all the experiments which I have performed upon the *glosso-pharyngeal nerve*, I am inclined to draw the following conclusions :

1. That this is a nerve of *common sensation*, as indicated by the unequivocal expression of pain by the animal, when the nerve is pricked, pinched, or cut.

---

* Appendix, B.
† Edinburgh Med. and Surg. Jour. 1838.

2. That mechanical or chemical irritation of this nerve before it has given off its pharyngeal branches, or of any of these branches individually is followed by extensive *muscular movements* of the throat and lower part of the face.

3. That the muscular movements thus excited, depend, not upon any influence extending downwards along the branches of the nerve to the muscles moved, but upon a *reflex action,* transmitted through the central organs of the nervous system.

4. That these *pharyngeal branches of the glosso-pharyngeal* possess endowments connected with the *peculiar sensations* of the mucous membranes upon which they are distributed, though we cannot pretend to say positively in what they consist.

5. That this cannot be the sole nerve upon which all other sensations depend, since the perfect division of the trunk of the nerve on both sides does not interfere with the perfect performance of the *function of deglutition.*

6. That the mechanical or chemical irritation of the nerve, immediately after the animal has been killed, is not followed by any *muscular movements,* when sufficient care has been taken to insulate it from the *pharyngeal branch of the par vagum.* And we here again observe an important difference between the movements excited by irritation of the *glosso-pharyngeal* and those of a motor nerve. For while the movements produced by the irritation of the *glosso-pharyngeal* are arrested as soon as the functions of the central organs of the nervous system have ceased, those from irritation of a motor nerve, such as the *pharyngeal branch of the par vagum,* continue for some time after this, and when all connection between it and the *medulla ablongata* has been cut off

7. That after perfect section of the nerve on both

sides, the *sense of taste* is sufficiently acute to enable the animal readily to recognize bitter substances.

8. That it probably may participate with the other nerves in the performance of the function of taste, but it certainly is not the special nerve of that sense.

Lastly, the *sensation of thirst,* which is referred to the *fauces* and *pharynx,* does not appear to depend entirely upon the presence of this nerve. The animals in which it was divided lapped water of their own accord. I observed one of them in which the nerves were found satisfactorily divided, rise, though very feeble, walk up to a dish containing water, lap some of it, and return again to the straw upon which he was previously lying."

Tenth Pair : — Pneumo Gastric or Par Vagum. — This nerve is unquestionably one of the most interesting and important of the nerves of the body. Its diseases are of the most alarming character, affecting digestion and respiration. It is a compound nerve, that is, it consists of two tracts of nervous matter bound up together, the one for sensation, the other for motion.

Solly says that both branches arise from the olivary bodies, as I have already quoted, when speaking of the medulla oblongata. Swan says they arise from the restiform body by the side of the groove between it and the olivary body just below the origin of the glosso-pharyngeal.

Its direction is outwards and forwards, and it passes out of the cranium by the foramen lacerum posterior, and descends with the sympathetic on the outer side of the external carotid artery, and passes into the chest, and in its course furnishes branches to the muscles of the pharynx and larynx, and by a superior and also an inferior or recurrent branch to the œsophagus, and then the cardiac, pulmonary, and gastric branches for the heart, lungs, and stomach.

From this distribution of the branches of this nerve we may infer that its functions are important. Let us inquire what they are?

Mr. Bell considers the pneumo gastric a respiratory nerve, and that it has a common origin with the respiratory nerves by the medulla oblongata, and goes to the larynx, lungs, heart, and stomach, and thus associates the muscular apparatus of respiration. He says the division of the recurrent branch destroys the voice, and if the laryngeal is divided this stops the connection between the muscles of the glottis and those of the chest, and that injury or compression of the pneumogastric produces difficulty of breathing. He thinks it may not be essential to the stomach, as it does not exist in animals without heart or lungs.

From numerous and careful experiments made by Dr. Reid, already alluded to, on the different branches of the par vagum, it appears that the pharyngeal branch of this nerve is the motor nerve of the constrictor muscles of the pharynx and the muscles of the soft palate ; and that the functions of the laryngeal branches are as follows:

1. "That the superior laryngeal furnishes one muscle only with *motor* filaments, viz. the crico-thyroid.

2. That the superior laryngeal furnishes all, or at least nearly all, the *sensitive* filaments of the *larynx*, and also some of those distributed upon the *mucous surface* of the pharynx.

3 That the inferior laryngeal or recurrent furnishes the *sensitive* filaments to the upper part of the trachea, a few to the *mucous surface* of the pharynx, and still fewer to the *mucous surface* of the larynx.

4. That when any irritation is applied to the mucous membrane of the larynx in the healthy state, this does

15*

not excite the contraction of the muscles which move the arytenoid cartilages by acting *directly* upon these through the mucous membrane, but this contraction takes place by a *reflex action*, in the performance of which the superior laryngeal is the *sensitive*, and the inferior laryngeal the *motor* nerve."

From other experiments to ascertain the functions of the œsophageal branches, it appears that section of the par vagum arrested the movements of the œsophagus, and paralysed its muscles, but he says :

" This arrestment of the movements of the muscular fibres of the *œsophagus* in deglutition after section of the *pneumogastrics*, does not depend upon any diminution in the contractility of the muscular fibres, but upon a breach being made in the nervous circle, which, through the intervention of the *medulla oblongata*, connects the muscular with the mucous coat. We, therefore, conclude that the muscular contractions of the œsophagus are not called into action by the ingesta acting directly as an excitant upon the muscular fibres through the mucous membrane, but by a reflex action, part of the *œsophageal* filaments of the *par vagum*, acting as a motor, and others in the manner of sensitive nerves. Or, to use the phraseology of Dr. M. Hall, the contraction of the œsophagus in deglutition is an excito-motory action — the filaments of the œsophageal nerves distributed in the mucous coat being the excitors, and those in the muscular coats being the reflex or motors."

From other experiments by the same gentleman to determine the influence of the cardiac branches upon the heart, it was ascertained that section of the par vagum above the oirgin of these branches does not materially affect the heart's action. But he thinks severe injury of the brain or even mental emotion, affect the contraction of this organ, probably through the influence of the par vagum, as he found by removing portions of each par vagum in rabbits, and then crushing the brain, the action of the heart was not increased and enfeebled as in rabbits whose heads were thus injured, but in whom the par vagum was entire.

He also found, by experiments to ascertain the influence of this nerve on the lungs, that division of one par vagum had no particular effect upon animals, even when sufficient was removed to prevent reunion. Division of both did not annihilate the want of fresh air in the lungs, the "besoin de respirer," as Brachet supposed, but the "division of both pneumogastrics," he says, "invariably proves fatal if the cut ends of the nerves are kept apart. The animal seldom if ever lives beyond three days, and generally dies sooner ; but when the cut ends of the nerves are allowed to remain in contact, it sometimes lives ten or twelve days. There can be no doubt that the section of these nerves proves fatal by its effects upon the lungs. The congested state of the blood-vessels of the lungs, and the effusion of frothy serum in the air-cells and bronchial tubes, may be considered as the characteristic and only constant appearance after death from section of the pneumogastrics."

The influence of this nerve upon digestion is well known, as division and separation of the cut ends of this nerve arrests digestion, though the mode in which this is produced is not well established, whether it is by producing paralysis of the muscular contractions of the stomach, or by arresting the secretion of the gastric juice.

This matter remains in uncertainty, though it is probable that only the muscular contractions of the stomach are under the guidance of the par vagum, while other actions, such as nutrition, secretion and absorption are under the influence of the great sympathetic. We also know that any dimunition of the nervous influence, as section of the medulla spinalis or injury of the brain stops digestion.

What light has pathology thrown upon this subject? Numerous cases are on record of tumors pressing on this nerve, causing great difficulty of breathing. Andral has published a case of severe dyspnœa, which seemed to be wholly produced by compression of the par vagum by a tumor in the neck. Blandin relates a case of a tumor in the nerve itself, which caused difficulty of breathing and symptoms of angina pectoris.

This nerve is also the seat of neuralgia, arising from irritation of this nerve, and giving rise to convulsive and periodical coughs, spasmodic asthmas, and spasms of the stomach, and nervous vomitings, &c.

M. Jolly has published several cases of this kind in the Nouvelle Bibliotheque Medicale for 1826, and I presume they are much more frequent than are suspected. The following is a case. A female, forty years of age, had long been affected with severe paroxysms of cough, resembling hooping cough, and which came on every evening after eating. It was attended by vomiting and convulsive agitation. Bleeding, purging, &c. were of no avail, and she was cured by tonics and anodynes.

M. Gendin relates a case of convulsive cough, produced by a wound in the neck, with loss of substance, which exposed this nerve to irritation.

Prof. Albers, of Bonn, found the par vagum unusually large in fifteen cases of phthisis pulmonalis. Intermittant croup appears to arise from affections of this nerve, as the following cases show.

CASE XLVII.— *Recurrent Dyspnœa.*— *Death.*— *Disease of a par Vagum.* — A man, twenty-four years of age, had for a length of time suffered from most distressing dyspnœa ; the respiration was always short, hurried, and confused, and to appearances was affected by the action of the thoracic muscles alone, the lungs being merely passive ; the horizontal position was quite intolerable ; the face was bloated ; the lips and alæ nasi of a livid hue ; the eyelids œdematous. No sign of any disease of the heart could be detected by the stethoscope. During a paroxysm of severe dyspnœa, this patient suddenly expired.

On dissection, a portion of the left par vagum was found quite enveloped in a mass of tuberculous glands, and the substance of the nerve itself was extremely indurated.

CASE XLVIII. — *Dyspnœa — Remarkable slowness of the pulse — Death — Disease of the Nervi Vagi.* — Maria Cocchi, aged forty, had enjoyed good health till her thirtieth year, when she had a severe attack of pneumonia : from that period the breathing had been always oppressed.

In October, 1832, having fatigued herself more than usual, had taken rather more wine than she had been accustomed to, she was seized with a stupor, which lasted for several days, and during which she was scarcely conscious. On recovering from this attack, the respiration was more difficult than ever, and the pulse which was naturally slow, became extraordinarily so, beating only twenty-four times in the minute.

The chest being carefully examined with the stethoscope, the respiratory murmur was heard over every part ; it was rather puerile : the sounds of the heart were regular, somewhat stronger, and might be heard over a greater extent than in health : the inference therefore was, that there was dilatation with hypertrophy of this organ. The diagnosis was certainly puzzling. A variety of remedies was tried, but with no good effect. Before death, the breathing became stertorous, and the face as purple as if she had been strangled.

Dissection. — The head was examined, but no decidedly morbid appearances found there. In the chest there were several recent pleuritic adhesions : the principal bronchial glands were greatly enlarged and loaded with a calculous matter : a considerable quantity of a yellow colored serum in the pleuræ, and also in the pericardium ; the texture of the heart quite sound, but its volume somewhat enlarged : a few patches of steatomatous degeneration were seen on the aorta : the pneumogastric nerves, a little below the larynx, were found imbedded in a mass of swollen glands, and these enveloped in cellular membrane, which was much loaded with blood : the right nerve seemed to have been most affected, and at one point it presented the appearance of having been " tiraille " and flattened.*

The learned and ingenious Dr. Hugh Ley, it is well known attributes Laryngismus Stridulus,† &c., to enlarged glands pressing upon this nerve or its branches, and the cases quoted seem to confirm his views.

It has been remarked that the corpus olivare appears to be the appropriate ganglia of this nerve. The following case from M. Jolly supports this opinion. A man had a series of anomalous symptoms, attributed by his medical advisers to some organic disease of the chest. The least

---

* Medico Chirurgical Review, vol. 22, quoted from Rust's Magazine.
† An Essay on the Laryngismus Stridulus, or Croup-like Inspiration of Infants. To which are appended, Illustrations of the General Principles of the Pathology of Nerves, and of the Functions and Diseases of the Par Vagum and its principal Branches. By Hugh Ley, M. D., &c., &c.

exertion of body or least mental emotion produced palpitation of the heart and tendency to suffocation. He was bled and starved, and died of general dropsy. The *only* morbid appearance was softening and vascularity about the corpora olivaria, at the origin of the par vagum.

I believe affections of this nerve are not uncommon, but are very frequently overlooked ; and, therefore, with the hope of attracting attention to this subject, I subjoin the following most interesting case from Dr. James Johnson.*

CASE XLIX. — "*Singular Case of Periodical Monomania, terminating in Suicide, with the Appearances on Dissection. By James Johnson, M D.*

" I think I may venture to assert that there is not a more remarkable — perhaps a more interesting case in the annals of medicine, than the following.

" Mr. M'Kerrell, aged about 56 or 7, had spent nearly thirty years in the civil service of the East India Company, and had risen to a high rank on the Madras establishment. He returned home about six or seven years ago, with an ample fortune. He was a gentleman of highly cultivated mind, and great natural abilities. He had suffered some severe attacks of fever in India ; but arrived in his native land with a comparative sound constitution. He had made some excursions to the continent, more for amusement than health, and, about four years previous to his death, had sustained an unsuccessful contest for the representation of Paisley. In this contest he went through an immense exertion of body, and excitement of mind. He dated his chief bodily and mental afflictions from this period. His digestive organs be-

* Medico Chirurgical Review, 1837.

came considerably deranged, and constipation of the bowels was a prominent feature of the malady, up to the very day of his death — which was occasioned by his own act. Very soon after the contest alluded to, he came under my care, and continued to consult me, with longer or shorter intervals, till the final and melancholy termination of his existence. At first, his corporeal ailments were alone referred to, and these were the common symptoms described by the generality of dyspeptics. There was an appearance in his manner, however, which led me to suspect some grievance kept in the back ground. The patient, being a man of great intelligence and knowledge of the world, he frequently detained me in conversations and discussions quite foreign to the objects of my visit, and dismissed me without entering upon them at all. One day he appeared more than usually depressed, and, after some ordinary conversation, he remarked that he thought me a man in whom he could confide, and who would not devulge a secret, if a pledge of secrecy were given. I observed, a little jocularly, that doctors were like priests, and confessions were held as secret by the physicians of the body as of the mind. But I observed, at the same time, that I had no wish or curiosity to become acquainted with secrets unconnected with my professional avocations. ' That,' said he, ' I believe ; but this is a secret directly connected with my health and happiness ; and I think its disclosure to a man of honor, and professional experience, might probably enable him to relieve me. But I had rather suffer the miseries which I endure, than confide the CAUSE of them to a physician who would divulge it.' In that case, I readily pledged myself to secrecy, provided there was nothing in the secret of a criminal nature, and which the laws of God or man did not call upon me to make known, if necessary. He answered, ' if you find in this secret any thing criminal, I absolve you from your promise.' I then pledged myself.

"It was with great difficulty, and tedious circumvolution, that he came to the point, being apparently tortured with shame in the disclosure. At length it came out that he labored under an illusion, which came on regularly every second day, and lasted till he went to sleep. He would awake the next morning free from the hallucination, and perfectly convinced that it was an illusion under which he had labored on the preceding day. At a later period, he often assured me that he was conscious of the illusion *being such*, and not a reality, on the days of its occurrence, though I have strong reason to suspect this statement, for up to the day of his death, he never would see me on the day of the illusion. The illusion itself let in no light on the nature of the complaint, and therefore the secret may be kept without any detriment to the history of this extraordinary case. Unfortunately, the entity in which it consisted, presented itself so frequently, and was mixed up with so many other objects and subjects, that he could not walk a street without seeing it, unless he kept his eyes shut ; he could scarcely read a page of a book without its crossing his sight ; he could hardly, indeed, survey the furniture and other things in his room, without being reminded of this torturing illusion. His sufferings were of two kinds ; one, directly connected with the illusion itself, which, according to his conviction, on alternate days, exercised a hostile influence on him, and was, as it were, an evil star, blasting every thing belonging to him by its malign radiation ! The other, was an indescribable horror, terror, or sense of destruction, having no direct reference to the illusion, and a degree of which continued after the delusion vanished, that is to say, during the ' good days.' This was a part of the complaint which appeared, both to the patient and

16

physician, as purely corporeal, the result of some disordered function or structure of the body. The illusion; on the other hand, had greater reference to the mental functions, though probably they were both the result of the same cause.

" I made numerous and minute examinations of the general health, without being able to detect any palpable cause for these strange phenomena. In respect to the head, this gentleman was highly gifted in intellectual powers, and his mind amply stored with varied and extensive information. He never displayed the slightest aberration, or even weakness of mind, except as regarded the hallucination; and even *that* he regarded in its true light, when the mental cloud had passed away. There was no physical symptom of any cerebral or spinal affection. The senses and sensibility were perfect, as were all the muscular powers. He was, however, emaciated, and the emaciation gradually, though slowly, increased.

" I frequently examined the chest, and it sounded well, in all parts ; the patient could expand it freely ; and he could take great exercise without any shortness of breath. He had no cough. The pulse was remarkably small, and generally slow. I confess that, at no period of my professional attendance, which lasted three years and a half, did I suspect any disease of the heart or lungs, though in both cases, I was mistaken, as the final event proved.

" In respect to the abdominal viscera, there were many symptoms of disordered digestion, but none of organic disease. He ate two meals of animal food.daily, the aggregate being considerably more than a man in health, and using but moderate exercise, would naturally consume. The patient found it necessary to confine himself almost entirely to plain animal food, with bread, and very little wine, or weak brandy and water. Any deviation from this system occasioned considerable inconvenience, both as to the common symptoms of indigestion, and also as respected the main and permanent malady. The constipation of bowels, as before remarked, was very obstinate, and the fæces were generally in the form of scybala, even when aperients were employed. All strong or drastic purgatives aggravated his complaints. The functions of the kidneys were very rarely disturbed. Thus, then, repeated examinations of the various organs, through the medium of their functions, disclosed to me no tangible or cognizable proof of structural disease. Yet such disease did actually exist, however humiliating may be the confession. This does not militate against the science of medicine, but only against my own powers of discrimination.

"The regular, the unerring periodicity of the main symptoms, puzzled me not a little; and this periodicity I could not help attributing to some physical, rather than to a moral cause. What tended to embarrass me still more was the fact that, on the ' good day,' he could view the ENTITY, whether simple, or in any of its combinations, with composure, while on the ' bad day,' or the day on which the illusion was in the ascendant, the sufferings which this unfortunate, and highly-gifted individual experienced, were such, that the narration of them often rendered me, as it were, a participator of his miseries, and deprived me of sleep. I can conscientiously say that I heartily repented of being the depositary of the secret, and the physician of the patient.

"In the early part of the year 1834, while in Scotland, Mr. M'Kerrell was suddenly seized with hæmoptysis, though not to any extent; and some of the most respectable medical practitioners of Edinburgh were consulted. I may mention Dr. Abercrombie, the late Mr.

Turner, and Mr. Scott. The complaint subsided without any serious consequences; though there were a few very insignificant returns of it afterwards, for which I attended the patient in the succeeding year — 1835.

" And now I suddenly lost sight of him, and knew not whether he had directed his steps. On the 15th of November, I was summoned to him, and found him considerably altered in appearance. Although it was the 'good day,' he was evidently laboring under great mental depression and distress. He stated that he had been some time at Cheltenham, and had consulted an old and valued friend, who prescribed for him, but in vain, as his mental and corporeal miseries were now arrived at a degree of intensity, which human patience could not long bear, nor human strength resist. He had got much thinner, and complained that some aperient medicines which he had been taking at Cheltenham, increased rather than diminished his sufferings. This, however, was probably imaginary.

" The remainder of the tragic scene is well known to the public. When I parted from him on the 15th of November, being his 'good day,' though a very wretched one, he desired me to call again on the 25th of the same month, which would also be his 'good day,' On Tuesday, the 24th, however, being the day of the illusion, he wrote a short letter to Mrs. Vickery, his landlady, announcing his determination to commit suicide, and giving her some directions about his keys, and the place of his sepulture. He rang the bell about four o'clock, and ordered a wine-glass. At a quarter before seven o'clock, he was found lying on the floor, dead, and nearly cold with an empty two-ounce phial labelled ' hydrocyanic acid,' of Scheele's strength, on the table, standing beside the empty wine-glass. In the bottle, there was a drop or two of the acid, exhaling the odor of almonds !

"*Dissection,* 27 *hours after Death.* — The body was examined by Mr. Henry Johnson (my son), and Mr. Bushel, in presence of Dr. Robert Lee, Mr. Harding, and myself.

" The emaciation was very great. The deceased having fallen on his face, there were marks of contusion about the temple, and the face itself was rather of a bluish hue. The body exhaled an odor of Prussic acid. The eye did not present any particular appearance. The stomach was remarkably capacious, and its contents were sent to Dr. Turner, for analysis. In some portions of the mucous membrane of this organ, especially near the upper and inferior orifices, there were marks of recent inflammation, particularly in stellated patches, where slight marks of extravasation were perceptible. In several portions of the small intestines, the external hue was dark, almost approaching to livid ; and the mucous membrane of these portions was vividly red, or of a dark red color ; but without extravation, or perceptible injection of the vessels. It resembled imbibition, or that which would be produced by steeping sound, yet dead parts, in blood. The large intestines were greatly distended by air, but exhibited no marks of disease of any kind.

" The liver, spleen, mesentry, kidneys, and all the abdominal viscera, were perfectly sound.

" Before a knife was laid on the body, I expressed a wish that the ganglionic centres might be carefully examined, as I conceived that some irritation of the nerves of organic life played an important part in the phenomena exhibited by the patient. The solar plexus was therefore minutely investigated ; but nothing abnormal was perceptible.

" In the thorax there was great and varied disease. The lungs were studded with tubercles, especially the superior lobes, and extensive adhesions existed between

16*

the pleuræ-costales and the p. pulmonales. None of the
tubercles had broken down, so as to discharge their contents through the bronchial tubes.

"The heart was not larger than natural, or very little
more than the ordinary size ; but the pericardium was
universally adherent, by old, that is to say, by cellular
attachments. The organ itself presented one of the fin-
est specimens of 'simple hypertrophy,' which we have
ever seen. The parietes of the left ventricles were an
inch and a quarter in thickness ; and the cavity was,
with difficulty, discovered. It could not have contained
more than four drachms of blood, if so much ; which is
scarcely one-third of that which a normal ventricle
would be capable of throwing out at each contraction.
There was nothing abnormal in the arteries. The blood
in every part of the body was perfectly fluid, and exhibited not a single coagulum in any vessel.

"The brain was remarkably firm, and the vessels were
rather congested ; but there was no visible trace of disease in the head. The skull was of unusual thickness
and density.

"And now comes the most remarkable portion of the
pathology. Upon the nervus vagus, or pneumo-gastric
nerve of the left side, just before the recurrent is given
off, there was affixed a hard jagged body, the size of a
kidney-bean, or small nut, composed of calcareous matter, and probably a diseased bronchial gland converted
into this substance. The union of the nerve and this
rugged mass was so intimate, that no dissection, without
cutting the nerve or the calcareous body itself, could
separate them. The foreign body, in fact, had penetrated, or at least invaded the nerve, which was thickened
at this part. Lower down, and involving the cardiac,
pulmonic, and œsophageal plexuses in a labyrinth of per-
plexity, were several diseased bronchial glands, render-

ing the dissection a tedious and difficult operation. The parts were all carefully removed, and the investigation conducted slowly, and at different periods, in the Kinnerton-street Theatre of Anatomy, by Mr. Johnson, Mr. Tatum, Mr. C. Johnson, and others. The preparation is preserved in the museum, and may be seen by any gentleman there.

" When we consider that the nervus vagus rises in the medulla oblongata, but is chiefly distributed to the great organs *not* under our control, and that it communicates with almost the whole of the ganglionic nerves, we may form some idea of the irritation and disturbance produced in the digestive, sanguiferous, and sanguific organs, by a jagged calcareous mass, implanted, as it were, into one of the most important nerves of the great vital viscera ! "

Eleventh Pair : — Lingual or Hyo-Glossal, Arises from the pyramidal body half an inch below the origin of the sixth pair, and goes to the muscles of the tongue, and to those of the os-hyoides.

Experiments by Mayo and Fodera show that this is a nerve of motion only, and pathology supports this conclusion.

When irritated in an animal recently killed, the tongue becomes convulsed, and when both are divided it becomes motionless.

Twelfth Pair : — Spinal Accessory. — Mr. Bell, calls this the superior respiratory nerve. It arises from the cervical portion of the spinal marrow, commencing opposite the sixth or seventh cervical vertebrae, passes upwards and enters the skull and joins the pneumogastric, and passes from the skull in the same sheath with this nerve. In passing through the foramen lacerum, it divides into two branches, an internal and external. The internal, after giving off some filaments to assist in forming the pharyngeal branch of the *par vagum*, becomes incorporated with the filaments of the trunk of the *nervus vagus*. The *external branch* proceeds outwards, perforates the upper part of the *sterno cleido-mastoideus*, sends filaments to this muscle, and to the *trapezius*, and forms at the same time several anastomoses with branches from the *cervical plexus*.

Dr. Reid already quoted, thinks from his experiments that it is not as Mr. Bell supposes a nerve of respiration. He states "that the *sterno cleido-mastoideus* and *trapezius* can assist in the involuntary movements of respiration after section of the *spinal accessory*, and therefore it cannot be called the special respiratory nerve of these muscles. As far as we can observe, the functions of the external branch of the *spinal accessory* resemble those of the filaments coming from the *cervical plexus* with which it anastomoses so freely."

"That the internal branch of the spinal accessory assists in moving the muscles of the pharynx we are satisfied, not only from the experiments just stated, but also from those upon the pharyngeal branch of the *par vagum*. Of the probable destination and functions of the other filaments of the *internal* branch of the *accessory*, we cannot pretend to judge without more extended inquiries. We certainly do not consider that these experiments entitle us to assert that they are not motor filaments.*"

---

* The dissection of Bendz, to which we have already referred, seem to show that these filaments of the accessory are distributed upon the larynx and œsophagus. They therefore probably assist in the movements of these parts.

SECTION V.

GREAT SYMPATHETIC NERVE.

The great sympathetic, trisplanchnic, ganglionic, great intercostal, are names given to a system of nerves, composed of a series of ganglions connected to each other by means of intermediary filaments, and of a few longer and larger cords. This system of nerves appears to be first formed and coeval with the *punctum saliens.* It extends from the base of the cranium down the side of the spine to the coccyx, and communicates by means of small filaments with the spinal nerves, and with several of the cerebral. The ganglions are irregular in shape, but generally roundish and of a reddish grey color, and seem to be made up of a network of numerous fasciculi, enveloped in a double coat of cellular membrane. At its upper part, when concealed in the carotid canal, the Great Sympathetic has the appearance of a ganglionic plexus, sending off some small branches, two of which join or entwine around the sixth cerebral nerve, and another communicates with the Vidian branch of the fifth nerve. The opthalmic, the spheno-palatine, and maxillary ganglions, are by some classed among those of the great sympathetic. Passing down each side of the spine, it presents many ganglions, viz.

3 in the neck,   called Cervical.
12 " " back,   "   Thoracic.
5 " " lumbar region, "   Lumbar.
3 or 4 " " sacral region, "   Sacral.

From these ganglions numerous filaments are given off, which interlace and form plexuses. Some filaments from the cervical and thoracic thus interlace and form the *cardiac plexus*, from which the nerves of the heart proceed, a branch also goes to each intercostal artery from the thoracic ganglion. From the fifth, sixth, seventh, eighth and ninth of these ganglions proceeds the great splanchnic or visceral nerve, which being joined by the lesser splanchnic nerve from the tenth thoracic ganglion, passes through the pillars of the diaphragm and terminates in a large plexus called the semilunar plexus or ganglion, and which lies partly on the aorta near the origin of the coelic and superior mesenteric arteries. This by uniting with its fellow and with other ganglia that are near constitute the *solar plexus*, or vast nervous network lying on the vertebral column, the aorta and crura of the diaphragm, and from which nervous filaments proceed, and accompany the arteries to all the viscera of the abdomen.

For further particulars respecting the anatomy of the great sympathetic, I refer the reader to Anatomical works.

It is known that this nerve accompanies the internal and external carotids, the basilic and the brachial arteries and the femoral; and it is generally believed by anatomists that filaments from it accompany all the arteries of the body to their ultimate distribution, and probably it is the source of the nervous power possessed by the capillaries. Weber observes that the muscular system is developed in proportion to the sympathetic nerve.

From the general distribution of this portion of the nervous system, it is evident that its functions are important, and deserving of the most careful study and investigation. But what the uses of this system of nerves are, has not been fully ascertained.

Some as Petit, Winslow, Bichat, Reid and others have considered the ganglions as nervous centres, independent of each other, but communicating with one another and with the brain and spinal marrow. While others as Chaussier consider the sympathetic as a cerebral nerve, and some as Le Gallois, Beclard, Lobstein, &c., believe it to be a spinal nerve.

Perhaps the most general opinion and the one entitled to most weight is that the ganglions are centres in which nervous power is developed, that they remove the parts they furnish with nervous energy, from the empire of the will, that these centres are however subordinate to the great cerebro-spinal system and do not prevent the transmission of strong impressions.

From the experiments of Brachet, who believes the great sympathetic constitutes an independent nervous system, it appears that this system presides over the contractions of the heart, and by dividing the cardiac plexus and all its filaments, the circulation which went on well before was instantly arrested. Fœtuses have come into the world well formed, but destitute of cerebrum, cerebellum, and medulla spinalis, hence the circulation must have been undisturbed. The ganglionic system in such was found perfectly well formed and well developed and according to Serres and others even more than in other fœtuses.

In Graefe and Walther's Journal is a case detailed by Prof. Meyer of Bonn, of the absence of the whole cerebro-spinal system. The being was a complete vegetable. No nervous filaments were to be found entering the muscles. The sciatic, crural, and obturator nerves were all wanting. It possessed however a ganglionic nervous system under the influence of which it must have grown.

It also appears from M. Brachet's experiments that chymification or secretion of the gastric juice wholly depends on the ganglionic system, though this system has no effect upon the contractions of the stomach, as these probably depend on the pneumogastric. It also appear that the other secretions, absorption, exhalation, genera tion and conception are dependent upon the ganglionic system. We know that in injuries of the spinal cord which paralyse the lower extremities and the rectum and bladder, both as to motion and sensation, that secretion, exhalation and absorption continue, showing that they are not dependant upon the cerebro-spinal system.

What further light has pathology thrown upon the functions of the ganglionic system? I regret to say that examinations of the condition of this system after death, have been too much neglected. Often, when most of the organs of the body are examined with great care, the great sympathetic and its ganglions are entirely overlooked.

Professor Lobstein, who has given much attention to the functions and diseases of the great sympathetic, believes that Hypochondriasis, Hysteria, Angina Pectoris, Lead Colic, and Incubus arise from a morbid condition of this nerve. We believe that physicians are very generally of the same opinion as regards most of the above diseases, and also that numerous other nervous abdominal affections have the same origin.

Mr. Teale, already mentioned, thinks the ganglionic system is subject to disease, and that its affections produce Neuralgia of the heart and stomach, causing palpitations, flatulence, &c.

The following cases from Lobstein,* where examination after death exhibited disease of this system, are worthy of attention.

---

* De Nervi Sympathetici Humani Fabrica, &c.   Auctore J. F. Lobstein, &c.   Parisis, 1823.

CASE L. — "A female of regular habits, had suffered from spasmodic and hypochondriacal symptoms, from the age of puberty, and had twice been attacked with incomplete apoplexy, which left a slight paralysis of the right side of the face; at forty-two, she was married, and became pregnant fifteen months after. At the eighth week of utero-gestation, a train of symptoms arose which subjected the patient to great misery. She had vomiting to such an extent, that, for three months, she immediately rejected every thing taken into the stomach; no relief being afforded by any internal medicine or external application. During the last seven days of her life, even a drop of water, when swallowed, was refused by the stomach. The internal fauces and the mouth first became inflamed, and subsequently mortified, from the continued excitement of vomiting; and the patient's fingers, in consequence of her sometimes putting them into her mouth, were ulcerated by the acrid discharge. The most distressing symptom of all, however, was a burning pain along the course of the spine, and in the lower part of the right hypochondrium, by which a constant jactitation was produced, and the strength of the patient exhausted. The only means by which this pain could at all be alleviated, was dry friction, so that the skin was quite excoriated. The unfortunate patient at last died in a state of miserable extenuation. The body was examined forty-eight hours after death. Much attention was given to the brain, but no unnatural appearance of any kind discovered. The head was thought to be rather under the usual size, but the patient had not been deficient in mental endowments. The thoracic viscera were in a state equally sound; the stomach presented no organic lesion, although there had been black vomiting, neither did the rest of the alimentary canal, nor the urinary system, differ from their healthy condition. The liver was

17

soft and livid. The uterus, in the fifth month of pregna-
cy, shewed no marks of disease, except some fibrous
tumors in its substance, equalling walnuts in size. The
cervix uteri was hard, perfectly closed at its external
orifice, by which it had resisted the attempts made to
procure abortion, and thus get rid of the vomiting by removing its cause. The fœtus was healthy, and in its
natural situation. The viscera were now all removed,
and the semilunar ganglion cut out ; it was not, indeed,
converted into a foreign substance, but its color was intensely red, which was regarded as true and genuine
inflammation, by some men of experience, and great cul-
tivators of anatomy, to whom this observation was communicated. The inflammation was so obstinate. that the
ganglia were but little paler after three days' infusion in
cold water ; and I took care to have the right ganglion
drawn in this state, and represented in the seventh plate
of this treatise. Its upper part is of a vivid red, but the
inferior, from which the mesenteric branches go off, is
more livid. The splanchnic nerve appeared to me much
broader than usual, before its entry into the ganglion."

CASE LI. — " The body of a girl was examined, who
had been attacked with epidemic cough, which was converted by metastasis first into spasmodic vomiting, and
then into atonic convulsions, which could not be overcome by any remedial means. In this case the left portion of the solar plexus was inflamed ; the right being
healthy."

CASE LII. — " A man, aged forty-seven, had a fibro-
cartilaginous tumor, which adhered loosely to the spine,
cut out. In two years, he returned to the hospital, having another tumor on the same site ; he was seized with
tetanus, and died in two days. On opening the body,

were found, first, a vascular cyst well filled with blood, at the surface of the medulla spinalis, and a quantity of serum effused within the sac formed by the dura mater ; secondly, very distinct inflammation of the semilunar ganglia."

CASE LIII. — " In a boy of ten years old, who died with symptoms of anxiety and oppression in the chest, and rattling at the pit of the stomach, in consequence of the retrocession of an exanthematous eruption, the author found a part of *the sympathetic nerve inflamed, with phlogosis of the ninth and tenth thoracic ganglia, and two of the anastamosing branches* sent off from the costal nerves."

The effect of the division of the sympathetic nerve, in the neck, where it accompanies the par vagum, upon the eye, deserves notice. In a short time after this division, often very rapidly, the conjunctiva becomes red and swollen, projecting over the cornea. That it is the division of the sympathetic and not the par vagum that causes this, is evident from the fact, that the removal of the superior cervical ganglion of the sympathetic has the same effect.

This nerve and its ganglia have been found inflamed after death from severe accidents, in which the constitution sympathised with the injured part, as in severe burns. Its ganglia have been found inflamed in Tetanus, and some have supposed that this inflammation is the first link in the chain of morbid action, which produces Tetanus. But as the ganglia of the sympathetic have been found inflamed without any tetanic symptoms, we cannot regard this inflammation as essential to Tetanus. In numerous cases of Colica Pictonum, the ganglia of the sympathetic in the abdomen have been found in a morbid state, swollen and inflamed.

The same ganglia have been found inflamed after death,

from severe fevers.   Dr. Cartwright, in his Essay on the
Fever of Natches, states, that in all his dissections,
during the epidemic of 1823, he found the sympathetic
ganglia inflamed.

They were found in a morbid state in malignant Cholera.   Delpech* says : " The common and ordinary result has been a remarkable alteration, principally of the
semilunar ganglions.   Those organs are more voluminous, and of a texture less dense than the nerves of the
adjoining plexuses, have probably retained better the
traces of the physiological alterations which they have
experienced ; they have often shown themselves swollen,
red, more or less strongly injected, and sometimes softened to a very remarkable degree.   The injection which
penetrates them, colors them red, when in all the remainder of the body the capillary system is injected black.
This very remarkable phenomenon cannot fail to recall
the painful sensation which occurs so constantly in the
prodromes, and in the beginning of cholera, and the precise seat which it occupies.

" The solar plexus is likewise in an unnatural state,
which is more or less obvious, but always perceptible by
the size of the nerves which compose it, often by the
red injection of their neurilema, and sometimes even by
the softening of the nerves which form it, which are
then ruptured by the slightest effort, or the lightest pressure.   This plexus is then formed by broad red bands,
and not by filaments of a greyish white, as in the natural state.

" The renal plexuses have presented sometimes alterations of the same kind, but they have not showed themselves so frequently, and never with the same intensity.
The affection appears to have been a simple extension of
that of the adjoining nerves."

---

* Etude du Cholera Morbus en Angleterre et en Ecosse, p. 196.

We know but little, it is true, of the functions of the great sympathetic, but enough to convince us they are important, and, considering our deficiency of knowledge of its pathology, we cannot but lament its condition is so little regarded in disease and in post mortem examinations.

17*

Part II.

DISEASES OF THE BRAIN, AND OF OTHER PARTS OF THE NERVOUS SYSTEM.

INFLAMMATION OF THE BRAIN, AND OF ITS MEMBRANES.

It has already been remarked, that our knowledge at present, is not sufficient, to enable us to say confidently, what symptoms distinguish inflammation of the substance of the brain from that of its membranes, though some distinguished pathologists as Rostan, Lallemand, Bouillaud and others, conceive they can frequently decide from the symptoms whether the substance of the brain is affected or only its membranes, and even distinguish the different stages and degrees of inflammation. Fortunately these distinctions are not of very great practical importance.

From what has been already stated when treating of the pathology and functions of the brain, it is evident that inflammation of the membranes that cover the superior and anterior portions of the brain, and inflammation of the cortical substance are accompanied by delirium, and that of the base of the brain and its membranes by coma, and often without delirium. It is, however, quite rare for the inflammation to be confined wholly to either of these portions of the brain.

The inflammatory affections of the brain and its membranes are known by different names, such as Arachnitis or inflammation of the arachnoid membrane, Meningitis or inflammation of all the membranes, and Cerebritis or inflammation of the substance of the brain. Phrenitis is a general term used for all the forms of inflammation of the brain, and of its membranes, attended with frenzy or violent delirium.

Acute Hydrocephalus or dropsy of the brain, is but one of the forms by which inflammatory action of the brain terminates, the effusion being the consequence of the inflammation. The term is, however, deceptive and improper. It is not the water which is to be dreaded or which constitutes the disease, but the previous inflammatory action; if this is arrested no effusion takes place — if it is not, death ensues, and sometimes before effusion occurs.

Inflammation of the brain terminates not only by effusion but by suppuration — the formation of false membranes and by softening or ramollisement of the substance of the brain.

Though, as it has been said, it is impossible in many cases to determine from the symptoms what part of the brain is affected, yet in some I believe it is not. The duration of the disease is some guide to us. If a patient for a long time has severe and fixed pain of the head, slight confusion of ideas, partial loss of memory, dejected appearance and altered manner, with disturbance of some of the senses, followed by either paralysis, rigidity or contractions of the muscles or by convulsions; we may properly infer that the disease is in the deep seated parts of the brain, and probably of that form of disease which terminates in ramollisement of the brain, though this condition may be accompanied by suppuration or by extravasation of blood into the same organ.

Affections of particular senses or muscles, while others remain undisturbed and the mind clear, should lead us to infer organic disease confined to the base of the brain, and to the origin or course of the nerves of the affected sense or muscles.

Examples of such affections of the brain have already been given, from which it is evident we may not unfrequently determine from the symptoms the part of the brain diseased.

The most characteristic symptoms of the inflammatory affections of the head are, fever, pain of the head which the patient considers of an unusual kind, increased sensibility of the eye to light, and often of the ear to sound and the skin to the touch. Sleeplessness, frightful dreams, sickness of the stomach, vomiting, pain of the limbs, retraction of the head, convulsions and delirium.

In some cases convulsions are the first symptoms that attract attention. Generally, however, inflammatory affections of the brain in children are preceded by langour and indisposition to move, especially to hold the head down, irritable temper, startings in sleep, desire to be alone and away from the light. In one case which I saw and which proved fatal, that of a fine little girl nine years of age, so great was the inclination to be alone or away from the noise of the family, that for several evenings previous to her making any complaint, she was found sitting by herself out of doors. Often slight spasms about the muscles of the eye and face, and a staggering gait are noticed before any complaint is made. Such slight symptoms should awaken attention, and if accompanied by pain of the head, vomiting, impatience of light or noise and febrile symptoms, should lead us to immediate exertions to prevent serious disease.

The increase of inflammatory diseases of the brain of late years, is a subject to which I wish to direct attention, and I cannot more strikingly exhibit the fact of this increase than by referring to the *Report of the City Inspector of the Interments in the City and County of New York* for above thirty years, from the commencement of making returns of deaths to the City Inspector in 1804 to the year 1838.

From the tables of the deaths from different diseases it appears that while the population of New York has only quadrupled in the last thirty years, the deaths from inflammatory affections of the head, or from inflammation and Dropsy of the brain alone, has increased more than twelve fold.

In the six first years of this period the deaths from these two diseases, which may be regarded as identical, were as follows :—

	1805.	1806.	1807.	1808.	1809.	1810.
Inflam. of brain,	17	16	15	17	18	12
Dropsy do.	16	22	30	28	28	42

	1833.	1834.	1835.	1836.	1837.	1838.
Inflam. of brain,	101	120	150	159	161	155
Dropsy do.	305	347	382	268	365	368

The population of the City of New York has risen during this time as follows :—

1805	.	.	.	.	.	,	.	75.770
1810	.	.	.	.	.	.	.	96.373
1815	.	.	.	.	.	.	.	100.619
1820	.	.	.	.	.	.	.	123.706
1825	.	.	.	.	.	.	.	166.086
1830	.	.	.	.	.	.	.	197.112
1835	.	.	.	.	.	.	.	270.089

It will be perceived that the most alarming increase has been of Dropsy of the head, an inflammatory affection of the membranes of the brain and mostly confined to children.

It should also be noticed that other diseases of the brain such as Apoplexy, Epilepsy, Insanity and Convulsions, are not at any period included in the above tables; these are classed seperately.

I have examined the bills of mortality in other cities in this country and find that in all, there has been a vast increase of inflammatory diseases of the brain within the last half century.

It also appears that the same diseases have of late greatly increased in England and France.

According to the late Dr. Davis, of London, eight out of forty-five deaths, in the *Universal Dispensary* were produced by Dropsy of the brain, and Dr. Allison states that forty out of a hundred and twenty patients die of this disease in the *New Town Dispensary*, London. Marshall, in his Mortality of the Metropolis, London, from 1629 to 1831 says that since 1790 deaths from Dropsy of the brain have been on the increase and to an alarming extent, the number being for the last few years about 800 per annum.

Dr. Coindet says that 20,000 deaths annually occur from the same disease in France.

What are the causes of this recent increase of the inflammatory diseases of the brain? It will be seen from other parts of this work that other diseases of the brain and nervous system have also increased; but our present inquiry is respecting the increase of the purely inflammatory affections of the brain. This increase is mostly of that form of inflammation denominated Acute Hydrocephalus or Dropsy of the brain. What then are the causes of this disease? These, as enumerated by authors, are blows or other injuries of the head, intestinal irritation, dentition, suppressed evacuations, repelled eruptions, intense and long continued mental application,

Golis* thinks the mechanical agitation of the brain in large active children by running, jumping &c., is a very frequent cause. He says the disease has much increased of late, and attributes some of this to the less frequent eruptions on the heads of children than formerly.

It will be observed that many of these causes are not more operative now than formerly, and therefore do not account for the increase.

Some recent writers have attributed many cases to anxiety and mental agitation of the mother during pregnancy. Golis observes, " that in the year 1809 when our imperial city, (Vienna) was bombarded, most of the children who were born after this frightful catastrophe in about twenty or thirty days after birth were seized by convulsions and died. Within the cranium were found traces of inflammation, and in the ventricles of the brain effusion of lymph and serum." Pinel mentions that out of ninety-two children born after the blowing up of the Arsenal in London, in 1793, eight were affected with a species of aretinism and died before the expiration of the fifth year ; thirty-three languished through a miserable existence of from nine to ten months duration, sixteen died on coming into the world, and six were born with numerous fractures of the large bones.

Early intellectual culture is considered by some a cause of this disease. A late writer observes, " the present plan of education in which the intellectual powers are prematurely exercised, may be considered as one of the causes of the more frequent occurrence of this disease."†

I am of the opinion that much of this increase of dis-

---

* A treatise on the Hydrocephalus Acutus, by L. P. Golis. Translated from the German, by Robert Gooch, M. D., London.

† Medico Chirurgical Review, April, 1826.

eases of the brain in infancy and childhood, is to be attributed to a predisposition to disease of that organ derived from the mother, and to causes that too greatly excite and develope too early and too rapidly the cerebral organs. A tendency to disease of the brain may be given to the foetus in utero, either as we have seen by the mental agitation of the mother, or by inheriting from her a nervous temperament, or in other words a brain and nervous system so excitable that slight causes will disorder it. The mother who possesses an excitable nervous system, either inherited or acquired, whose mind is easily agitated, who has had much mental anxiety and excitement, whose brain has been developed disproportionably to the other organs of the body, imparts this predominance of the nervous system to her infant, and then during its infantile years, when its brain is rapidly evolving and much blood is sent to it, this organ readily, and from very slight causes becomes diseased.

A predisposition to disease of the brain may be inherited from either parent, though I believe it is much the more frequently from the mother in consequence of her mental agitation during pregnancy. It is not improbable, indeed it is supported by established facts, that striking peculiarities of character that distinguish one of a family from other members of it, are derived from this source.

" If a mother," says Dr. Macnish, " while pregnant, is subjected to annoyances which fret and irritate her, the offspring will run a strong risk of inheriting a temper, similar to that under which she herself labored during gestation. Rizzo was murdered in the presence of Queen Mary, then pregnant with James VI. This monarch had a constitutional timidity of temperament, and a great horror of a drawn sword ; nor can it be doubted that the state of his mother's mind, while she was *enceinte*, contributed to stamp upon him those peculiarities which distinguished him in so marked and discreditable a manner from all the rest of the line of Stuart."

Diseases of the brain are far more common among children remarkable for precocity of intellect and who have large heads. In such they are also more dangerous. But this predominance of the brain, which produces the precocity of the intellect and disposes the child to disease, is very often an inheritance from parents, one or both of whom, have cultivated the mind, or in other words exercised and developed the brain, at the expense of the other organs of the body.

I have not any doubt but diseases of the brain will still increase, if the physical education of youth, especially of females, continues to be neglected; if intellectual culture continues to be deemed by parents and instructors so essential that infancy and youth must be chiefly devoted to it, and bodily labor and exercise neglected as a part of education.

They will also increase if mothers are not particularly attentive to the preservation of their own health, especially during gestation. Through that interesting portion of their lives, one of their highest duties is, to habitually cultivate calmness of mind, and equanimity of temper. Instead of agitating themselves with the existing topics of the times, and visiting places where their feelings are likely to be strongly agitated, they should strive to find enjoyment and health in attention to their domestic duties, and in daily, but gentle exercise in the open air.

It is a truth which cannot be too often repeated, that nothing is more essential to the welfare of any country, than the preservation of the health of its fomales, and I am pleased to see by an increased attention to their physical education, that many have become convinced of the fact.

18

Prevention. — From the preceding views of some of the causes of this disease, it is evident that preventive measures will often be serviceable. Attention on the part of mothers to their own health will do something towards diminishing the predisposition to disease of the brain in their offspring. As much may be done by them, by watchful care of their children during the first years of infancy and childhood. Their chief efforts should be directed to developing and perfecting the physical powers of their offspring. This can rarely be accomplished if children are early confined at school, and attempts made to improve their minds and store their memories to the utmost extent. Some children, especially those that are quite robust and intellectually dull, may bear such treatment without much injury, but the generality will not. Those that submit the most readily to this course or who learn the most rapidly, whose minds are precocious and active, will be the most likely to be injured. The parents of such should be apprised that although this precocity of mind, is not disease, it is akin to it, and should lead them to relax their attempts at mental culture and devote themselves to the improvement of their bodies.

Sometimes this predisposition to disease of the brain as exhibited by mental precocity is manifested by several members of the same family, and child after child dies of Dropsy of the brain. In such cases the utmost care should be taken to prevent all excitement of mind and to cultivate the physical system. No attempts should be made to improve the intellect. The whole paraphernalia of exciting play things should be dispensed with, and instead of carrying them to this and that place, to amuse them and to excite their curiosity, they should be left to pick up knowledge and to find amusement for themselves in the kitchen and parlor and garden. In this way they will have sufficient exercise and develope harmoniously and naturally their physical powers.

Treatment. — I regret to say that remedial measures for the relief of inflammation of the brain, when it is fully established are seldom successful. This makes me the more desirous that attention should be given to the means of prevention. It appears to me that the medical profession are too neglectful on this subject.

Sometimes when there are indications of approaching inflammatory disease of the brain, remedial measures seem to be very serviceable. An active purgative with rest, seclusion from light and noise, with cold applications to the head, sometimes appear to prevent the development of dangerous diseases of the brain.

When inflammatory disease of the brain is fully indicated and fever is present, bleeding and cold applications, even of ice to the head and active purgatives should be resorted to immediately. When good leeches can be obtained, I prefer the application of a large number, to general bleeding. In some cases, especially those attended by convulsions, the spinal cord is more affected than the brain. In such, leeches should be applied on the course of the spine. In all cases of disease of the brain requiring active depletion, 1 prefer taking blood from the nape of the neck — from the hollow called the pit of the neck. In some attacks leeches should also be applied to the temples, behind the ears, and to the interior of the nose, so as to produce copious bleeding.

Mercury has been strongly recommended by some to be given in Hydrocephalus until salivation is produced, but it is very difficult to produce this effect in children, and from what I have seen I believe that mercurial medicines are only beneficial in this disease by their cathartic effects.

Blistering and pustulation are serviceable after the activity of the disease has been subdued by bleeding. Sometimes recovery seems to result from a spontaneous eruption, this should encourage us in the use of external irritation.

But though this active depletory treatment is requisite in many, if not most cases, yet I am well convinced that symptoms resembling those of acute Hydrocephalus are produced by too much depletion, and particularly by long continued purging with calomel. Cases of drowsiness, pain and heaviness of the head, accompanied by dilated pupil and coma, may arise from excessive depletion, and may be cured by nourishment — cordials and opiates, while they will prove fatal under an opposite course. The absence of heat and fever distinguishes these cases generally.

It appears to me that opiates are too much avoided in some of the diseases of children, and that irritation from these diseases being thus unchecked, produces disease of the brain. Sometimes irritation of the bowels or irritation from teething may be controlled by an opiate, and which if not thus quieted would lead to disease of the brain.

M. Foville, in the 'Dictionnaire de Medicine et de Chirurgie Pratiques,' has advanced a new method of procedure in the treatment of this fatal disease. He recommends recourse to the *trepan* in violent cases. He says that the brain, occupying the whole interior of the skull, and being enveloped in a solid case, does not as other parts of the body receive pressure from the atmosphere. Consequently when more blood than usual goes to the brain, pressure of its substance must occur, and often does to such a degree as to destroy life.

He states the well-known fact, that bleeding does not so fully relieve this pressure on the brain as it does other organs, unless aided by the pressure of the atmosphere. And we know that in animals bled to death, though the lungs and other organs are pale and free from blood, yet the brain still contains a large quantity. M. Foville refers to numerous cases in which the removal of large portions of the skull by wounds and blows and even by fire was unaccompanied by severe inflammation or other bad symptoms.

I am disposed to think this method deserves consideration and trial, considering the fatal tendency of the disease. I have often been surprised to notice that severe blows on the head which fractured the skull to such a degree as to make it necessary to remove considerable portions of it, have been followed by no bad consequences; while on the other hand, I have frequently known slight blows upon the head, which in some instances have not fractured the skull at all, and in others only the outer table, to be followed by inflammation and other alarming symptoms and death. I am therefore of opinion that an opening in the skull might be beneficial in such cases.

I might quote numerous cases in support of the opinion that when a portion of the cranium is removed, then depletion seems to be very serviceable in preventing and relieving inflammation of the brain. The following curious case from Wiseman* will suffice.

"A person was wounded near the *Vertex* by a puncture of a dagger. He sent for a Chirurgeon, who dressed his wound and cured it; during which the patient daily went abroad without any consideration of it. About

---

* Chirurgical Treatise, by Richard Wiseman, Sergeant and Chirurgeon, Second Edition, London, 1636.

the seventeenth day, towards the full moon, as he was coming home one morning, he felt his legs faulter, and before he was got up stairs into his chamber his tongue failed him. His friends and servants put him into bed, and sent for me. They declared to me how he had been wounded such a day, and the manner of his being seized with the *Paralysis.* I saw a necessity for laying open the hairy scalp, and offered to go away that I might send for some of my servants to help me. He apprehending that I was leaving him as deplorable, catched hold of me, and would have spoke to me, but could not. He made signs for pen, ink and paper, and endeavored to write, but could not form one letter. He then threw himself down in the bed, breathing out *Jes.* I prayed his patience, telling him I would return suddenly. But before I went, I let him blood ten ounces, and returned again within one hour, and we found he had lost the use of his arms. I considered the wound, and concluding a necessity of setting on a Trepan, I caused his head to be presently shaved, and a circular incision about the wound. Then raising up the hairy scalp, smooth off with my *Spatula,* I both saw and felt the bone, but could discover no fault in it. I dried up the blood with sponges dipped in vinegar, raised up the lips round with my *Spatula* from the bone, and with a fresh sponge having dried up the blood, I looked again under them; but could discover nothing ill in the bared *Cranium.* I then filled up the wound with dossils of dry lint, and applied a digestive *ex terebinth,* over the lips, embrocating the parts about *cum ol. ros.* and laid on a cataplasm *e farin. hord. flor. rubr. balaust. in vino rub* with *syr. de ros. sicc.* &c. That day Sr. *Fr. Pruj.* gave him a visit, and prescribed him a Clyster, Cordials, Juleps, and what else he thought necessary. The next day was full-moon, at which time the brain is thought to rise high, and the vessels are turgid : wherefore I deferred the setting on the Trepan, contenting myself with the letting him blood again. All this while he was in a fever, and deprived of his speech and limbs. The next morning, between 10 and 11 of the clock, in the presence of Sr. *Fr. Pr.* Sergeant *Pyle,* Mr. *Arris* and Mr. R. who thought himself concerned for his servant, and had first dressed him, I took off dressings and looked into the wound. We found no Fissure, however there was a necessity of perforating the *Cranium.* Wherefore without delay I began to work with the Trepan, which I much prefer before a Trephine, it being an instrument which doth its work lightly, and cutteth the bone equally, or how you please, without pressing so heavily upon the head, and is approved by all the Chirurgeons abroad, being much to be recommended before the Trephine. After I had bored the bone, and taken it out, I looked into the hole, and seeing the *Dura Mater* retaining its natural color, without matter or blood, I dressed it up with a Sindon dipped in *ol. ros.* with a little Resin warm. This way of dressing was objected against, as I expected ; but I dressed it up, and assured them that I would cure this patient without applying any other remedy to the *Dura Mater* than these two simple medicaments: but withal I was much unsatisfied in myself, that such grievous symptoms, as loss of speech and limbs, with a fever, should afflict the patient, and yet no depressed bone or fissure, nor ought of matter or *Sanies* appear upon the *Dura Mater.* This, I say, troubled me much, I fearing some other place, or that the blood lay putrified under the *Dura Mater.* But I dressed it up with a soft round Dossil next the Sindon, and the bone with *liniment. Arcei,* continued the Digestive to the lips of the wound, and applied an *empl. de beton mag.* over all, then laid him down in bed. Going presently out of his close room (where I was crowded

up with great lights burning near me) into the fresh air,
I presently burst out with a violent coughing of blood;
yet the next day I dressed the patient again, and found
his speech and limbs restored; but he was hot and his
pulse quick. I opened his wound, and finding all as well
as I could expect, I dressed up the *Dura Mater* again as
before, with the same Oil and Resin, and after I had
bound him up as is usual in these cases, I let him blood
ten ounces, and advised the repeating of Clysters, &c.,
as occasion should offer. The Physicians and Chirurgeons visited him no more after the first dressing; but I
retained the young Chirurgeon that had first dressed his
little wound, he dwelling near the patient. After three
or four days dressing, this wound digested, and all the
symptoms went off. Upon which consideration, I diminished the quantity of the *ol. ros.* and increased the Resin;
making good my word in curing him with those simple
medicaments; I deterging and incarning as firmly and
speedily this way as by any Sarcotic I ever used. While
the bones were casting off, I cicatrized the lips as hath
been set down in the preceding observations. Coming one day to dress him while the wound was cic-
atrizing, he being abroad, I substituted the young Chirurgeon in my place; yet I saw him dressed twice or thrice
afterwards. He was well cured and remaineth so to
this day."

APOPLEXY.

"Apoplexy," says a late writer, "is now infinitely
more prevalent than in primeval times." It consists
essentially in pressure on the brain, though this pressure
may be produced in various ways — by extreme fulness
and engorgement of the blood vessels, or by the
extravasation of serum or blood. Some cases have

been reported in which no morbid appearances were discovered on examination after death. Such cases I apprehend must be extremely rare.

An apoplectic attack is characterized by the loss of sensation, voluntary motion and intellect, while the respiration and the action of the heart continue. The respiration is, however, laborious, and generally stertorous, though in some cases it has been natural. The pulse is slow and full, especially at the commencement. In the latter stages it is small, feeble and intermittent.

It is rare that an attack of apoplexy occurs without premonitory symptoms, though these are often so transient and variable as not to be regarded, while the general health remains good. These premonitory symptoms are a sense of fulness in the head, giddiness, throbbing of the carotid arteries, ringing in the ears, head-ache, temporary loss of recollection, numbness in some part of the body, and partial paralysis.

Apoplexy is a disease of civilized life, and one to which men are more subject than women. For the most part it is the result of full or luxurious living, excesses in drinking, diet or mental excitement. It is rarely seen among the laboring population unconnected with excess in the use of alcoholic drinks. Blacks are less subject to it than whites. It prevails in cities more than in the country. The sedentary, the idle and the meditative, are said to be most prone to it. According to Pousant, Monks are quite liable to it.

The form of the body is said to predispose to Apoplexy, as a corpulent habit, short neck and large head. Probably this disease does most frequently occur in persons of this formation as most authors so state, yet I have seen it as often in persons of a different formation.

I fully agree with Dr. Cheyne who thinks that habits of life most strongly dispose to the disease. He says,

"I am persuaded there is so much more in the habits, than in either the original form or diathesis, that I venture to affirm that in nineteen cases out of twenty of those who die of apoplexy the disease might have been averted or postponed by temperance." And he adds, "the daily use of wine or spirits, even in what is considered a moderate quantity, will lead a man of a certain age and constitution to apoplexy as certainly as habitual intoxication."

That this is true to the extent expressed, I can hardly believe, though I have no doubt the daily use of wine does strongly dispose persons to this disease. I have recently seen a fatal case of apoplexy in a person aged 45, moderately spare, whose appearance did not indicate an apoplectic tendency, but who for the last fifteen years had been in the wine trade, and in the daily use of wine, but not in excessive quantity. He was originally from a country town, and all his nearest relatives, parents, uncles and brothers I know, and none of them ever exhibited any tendency to this disease.

Excess in diet will also cause it. I have known several attacks after a full dinner. Both Portal and Rochoux say that apoplexy is much less frequent in Paris since the practice of eating hearty suppers has been abandoned.

Extremes of weather as to temperature, especially extreme hot weather, violent passions, great mental excitement and other causes determining more blood than usual to the head, cause this disease. Hence we find it to occur most frequently in the hot days of summer. The summer of 1838 was unusually hot, and the number of deaths in the city of New York from apoplexy, during the hot months was greatly increased over that of preceding years.

That great mental excitement causes apoplexy is

evident from the fact, that numerous instances have occurred of celebrated statesmen, lawyers and clergymen being seized with it while engaged in their peculiar duties and making great mental efforts. Instances are also quite numerous of violent passions, as anger causing an attack. Such are to be found in Bonetus, Cheyne and other writers on apoplexy. I am inclined to believe that long continued and great mental exertion disposes to cerebral disease — thus we find that many of the most distinguished statesmen, lawyers and literary men who have died within the last quarter of a century have been attacked with some form of cerebral disease.

Pathology. — As I have said some very rare cases of apoplexy exhibit on dissection no morbid appearance of the brain, but generally there is found great engorgement of the blood vessels, extravasation of blood or effusion of serum. Extravasation of blood may take place in any part of the brain or on its exterior surface, but it is most frequently found in the corpus striatum or in the thalami nervorum opticorum. It may proceed from the arteries or the veins. The arteries in the striated bodies, the small branches in the base of the brain that proceed from the carotid and vertebral arteries, the communicating artery, the basilar artery, the internal carotid and the vessels of the Plexus Choroides have been found ruptured in apoplexy.

It has been supposed that sudden attacks of apoplexy attended by paralysis of one side, arose from extravasation of blood, and into the hemisphere opposite to the affected side ; and that apoplexy from effusion of serum is more insiduous — the symptoms of oppressed brain manifesting themselves but slowly. These are I believe often distinctive signs, but not uniformly so, as sometimes after sudden attacks, with hemiplegia, no extravasation of blood has been found, but effusion of serum or a very injected, turgid state of the blood vessels.

Prevention. — Apoplexy is a malady of so grave a character that methods of prevention should be earnestly sought for and persevered in, whenever there are any indications of its approach ; and, as it has been remarked, there are, not unfrequently, such indications. Preventive measures consist chiefly in avoiding every thing likely to excite the action of the heart or that hinder the free return of the blood from the head. The particular cause which disposes to apoplexy should be ascertained. If it consists in repelled eruptions or suppressed evacuations they should be restored. If the symptoms that indicate the approach of this disease are caused by too plenteous diet, by the use of stimulating drinks, the habits in these respects should be changed. If there is numbness of the limbs or any paralytic symptoms, bleeding and purgation should be resorted to. Often a seton or issue in the neck will long avert an attack.

Above all, those threatened with apoplexy should renounce all business that occasions anxiety of mind, or that requires much mental effort, should take daily exercise in the open air by riding or walking, confine themselves mostly to vegetable diet, abandon all stimulating drinks, and sleep and eat but little. They should be particularly careful during summer and not expose themselves to the hot sun.

Treatment. — When an attack supervenes, bleeding is the first and most important remedial measure. This not only lessens the circulation in the brain but favors absorption. In addition to prompt and copious bleeding from one or both arms, bleeding from the nose by incision in the pituitary membrane, where it covers the septum of the nose, is salutary. All constriction of the dress about the neck or chest should be removed, the head should be elevated and very cold water poured upon it from a heighth of five or six feet. Ice should also be applied at intervals to the head, stimulating injections administered, and soon as the patient is able to swallow, he should take a drop of croton oil every two hours until the bowels move.

Every thing likely to excite the brain should be prevented from disturbing the patient, such as light, noise, company and conversation.

I have recently witnessed a severe attack in a person whose age, habits, and form of body were such as to predispose to it — which was relieved by prompt bleeding from both arms — cupping the neck and temples — ice and ice-water to the head, stimulating injections and croton oil.

After recovering from an attack, the patient should be interdicted all intellectual excitement, and live the remainder of his life as devoid of care as possible. His diet should be of the plainest kind, and water his only drink. He should avoid the extremes of heat and cold — and guard against all impediment to the free return of blood from the head by omitting neckcloths, or else wearing them very loosely, and be careful not to hold his head downwards.

I am aware that bleeding in attacks of apoplexy has been deemed unnecessary and improper by some, and emetics and tonics recommended. Cases may occur where this course is proper, but I have never seen a case in which I supposed it would. In all the attacks which I have witnessed followed by recovery, bleeding had been resorted to — in all those that have proved fatal where an opportunity was afforded for examining the brain after death, extravasation of blood was found, and

19

to such an extent that recovery from any course of treatment could not be expected.

The following cases have occurred within a few weeks and will illustrate my views of practice.

Case LIV. — Mr. L. K., aged about 65, full habit, large head, short neck, having exposed himself more than usual for several hours to the heat of the sun, suddenly fell deprived of sensation and voluntary motion. This occurred about mid-day. He was seen immediately — bled freely from both arms, his feet put in hot water and mustard sinapisms applied. His head was kept elevated and ice-water poured upon it, and surrounded at intervals with bags of ice. He also had a stimulating injection administered, was cupped in the neck and on the temples and took in the course of the afternoon, four drops of Croton oil, which moved his bowels freely. He soon rallied a little, but remained nearly insensible during the day and night following, but gradually and completely recovered after a few days. In this instance it appeared to me at the time, and does now, that the immediate and active treatment saved the patient. He has since this attack, now three months, enjoyed good health.

Case LV. — Mr. T., aged about 45, had been deranged in mind for about twenty years, but otherwise in good health.

In July, 1839, immediately after supper, fell insensible, was placed on a bed, and bled copiously This did not relieve him and he expired in about four hours. I examined his head and found large extravasations of blood into the corpora striata which had penetrated by ragged openings into the ventricles.

There was also slight extravasation into the Pons Varolii. In this case there was no indication of an approaching attack, and after its occurrence probably no measures would have been of service. But the two cases for the first hour were very similar. In this last case the patient having been deranged for twenty years, I was surprised to find there were no adhesions of the membranes of the brain. The only appreciable change found in the brain was a very unusual hardness of the cortical portion. The outer part of it seemed like a dense membrane and could be pealed off from the inner, which was quite red.

EPILEPSY.

" Epilepsy," says Dr. Baillie, " has become much more frequent within the last twenty years than formerly." Though this disease has been witnessed from the most remote times, as we find accounts of it in ancient authors, yet it prevails but little among uncivilized nations to what it does in civilized and enlightened communities.

"Epilepsy," says a late traveller, " as well as Apoplexy, is nearly unknown among the Laplanders," and we believe it is among all barbarous tribes. Females are more frequently the subjects of this disease than males.

But though this disease has always been known, and much has been written respecting it, it is still one of the most obscure diseases which afflicts mankind. A paroxysm, or an Epileptic fit is most mysterious and unaccountable. A person apparently in perfect health suddenly falls to the ground in a state of complete insensibility. He neither sees nor hears nor is he conscious of the most powerful impressions. His muscles immediately become convulsed, and sometimes, those about the face especially, violently so. The eyes roll about, the

tongue is often thrust spasmodically forward while the
face is livid, the breathing embarrassed and there is foaming at the mouth. The pulse is small, irregular and
frequent. Little by little these symptoms abate, the
breathing becomes freer, the pulse fuller, and more regular, the countenance more composed and the patient
is disposed to sleep.

Sometimes the epileptic person has some warning of
an approaching fit, such as confusion or pain of the head,
dimness of sight, noise in the ears, giddiness, &c., and
sometimes by what is called an *aura* or a sensation like
a stream of cool air or subtile fluid ascending from the
lower extremities. When this sensation reaches the
head the patient becomes unconscious. In such cases a
tournaquet applied just above the part first affected, has
sometimes prevented an attack.

Often the attack occurs in the night, during sleep.
There is much difference in the violence of these attacks.
In some the convulsive struggles are exceedingly violent,
in others there are scarcely none at all, the attack consisting only in loss of consciousness for a short time.

Death sometimes occurs during a paroxysm, but not
often, and patients suffer from them through a long life.
In some cases years intervene between the attacks, but
usually only a few weeks.

Epilepsy is sometimes the precursor of insanity, and
usually has a tendency to impair the intellect, though
some epileptics possess their mental powers unimpaired
to very advanced age. I have seen several cases in
which the disease seemed to improve the intellect, at
least for a time. It is a disease which affects all ages,
though children and young persons about the period of
puberty are most subject to it.

The causes of an Epileptic fit are numerous, and in
some cases it is difficult to say from what it does origin-

ate. All strong affections of the mind, those that increase and those that diminish the action of the brain appear to produce it, such as joy, anger, grief and terror, the last frequently causes it. Suppressed evacuations, repelled eruptions, irritation of the bowels, worms, dentition and eating very heartily appear at times to give rise to it.

The use of alcoholic drinks is a very common cause A case is related of a person who received a fracture of the skull and ever afterwards was subject to attacks of Epilepsy if he indulged in alcoholic drink, but was wholly free from them so long as he abstained. In fact irritation in any part of the body may give rise to Epilepsy.

The proximate cause of Epilepsy is supposed to be situated in the brain, as sometimes it results from injury of that organ, and in those who die during a paroxysm, the brain is found engorged with blood.

In some who have long been subject to Epilepsy without mental disturbance, and who have died of other diseases, the brain on examination exhibited no unnatural appearance. In most cases of Epilepsy however, some organic affection of the brain, its membranes, or of the bones of the cranium have been observed, but these affections are, I apprehend, oftener the effect than the cause of Epilepsy.

In those Epileptics who exhibit disturbance of the intellect, some organic affection of the brain is always found. M. M Brouchet and Casauvielh have published a valuable work on Epilepsy in connection with Mental Alienation, in which they state that the result of their researches show that Epilepsy is the result of chronic inflammation of the white substance of the brain ; while mental alienation results from chronic inflammation of the cineritious or grey portion of the brain.

These opinions though supported by many facts, can-

19*

not as yet be considered established. Further researches
are necessary. The brain and nervous system of those
who die of Epilepsy, should be examined with great care
and whenever opportunity presents, should be compared
with similar parts of those who have never been affected
by the disease. Without this comparison slight variations of color and consistence, might not be observed.

As I have said, injury of the brain from external violence sometimes disposes to attacks of Epilepsy. A
depressed or carious portion of the skull by irritating the
brain will cause these attacks, and they have been prevented by trephining and removing the injured bone.

The following are instructive cases.

CASE LVI. — "*Case of Epilepsy cured by Trepan-
ning. By Henry Coates, of the Royal College of Sur-
geons in London, and Surgeon to the Salisbury Infirmary.*

" James Goddard, ætat. 33, a gentleman's coachman,
was admitted a patient into the Salisbury Infirmary,
July 28th, 1804. He stated, that about four years
before, he was driving his master's carriage under a
gateway, (not stooping sufficiently,) the crown of his
head struck against a beam ; this at the time was not
followed by any other symptoms, than a slight headache
for a few days, and an inconsiderable swelling of the part,
which soon subsided. Nothing occurred to remind him
of the accident, till, about a year afterwards, when a
small tumor appeared on the part on which he received
the bruise, which, (to use his own language,) continued
to swell without much pain, and at last burst. The
wound was afterwards dilated by a surgeon, and healed
with difficulty in about six months, and he says, that he
continued perfectly well for about six months afterwards, when he was attacked with an epileptic fit while
on the coach box ; and has since had repeated attacks of

them at intervals of from a week to a month. He now complains of extreme pain in his head, loss of vision of his left eye, numbness and coldness of the left side, particularly of the foot; his general health and appetite are otherwise tolerably good. On examining the scalp, I perceived several small puffy ulcerations about the centre of the coronal suture, which, on pressure, give him pain. He was directed to take some opening medicine.

"July 29th, the appearance of the scalp indicating some further disease, I determined to ascertain the state of the bone, for which purpose I made an incision of about three inches in length in an oblique direction, beginning an inch in front of the sagittal suture and running backwards. The bone at the anterior part of the incision was found roughened, and a portion of it about the size of a shilling, porous, with a sinus in the centre, which readily admitted a probe being passed to the dura mater.

"I now determined to remove the diseased portion of the bone, and applied a trephine, the crown of which was sufficiently large to include the whole of it. The operation was tedious from the extreme delicacy of the part, and care required in the use of the instrument. It was, however, completed without accident, and on extracting the bone, its internal surface had an honeycomb appearance. The dura mater was detached, but perfectly healthy.

"The wound healed kindly, and I have seen him several times lately; he continues well, and follows his usual occupation; he has had no return whatever of the fits. The numbness and coldness of his left side is quite removed. The vision of his left eye is better, though not quite recovered."*

CASE LVII. — " *Epilepsy of thirty-three Years' stand-ing, cured by the removal of a Carious portion of the Cranium.*

"One of the inmates of the Hopital des Invalides, 63 years of age had been wounded at the battle of Marengo with a piece of a small shell (obus) in the forehead. He was immediately trepanned, and a portion of the bone extracted. The symptoms of commotion and of com-pression were succeeded by those of encephalitis. When these subsided, he was found to be paralytic on the right side, and to have lost completely ' la memorie des choses.' The wound never fairly healed, but remained fistulous ; and scarcely a day passed over without an attack of epileptic convulsions. For the last thirty-three years, he had been in this deplorable condition, subjected to daily fits, totally deprived of his memory of things, and having a fistulous sore on his forehead. M. Larrey having de-tected with a probe a loose portion of bone, divided the integuments, and extracted it with a forceps. The wound and sore speedily healed up, the attacks of epilepsy have ceased to return, and his locomotive and mental faculties have become considerably improved. We are informed, however, that his memory of numbers and of names is still very imperfect and wavering. — *Lancette Francaise.*"

Tumours pressing upon and involving nerves some-times cause Epilepsy.

The following case is from the fourth volume of Med-ical Essays and Observations by a Society in Edinburgh, 1737.

CASE LVIII. — " *An Epilepsy from an uncommon cause ; by Dr. Thomas Short, Physician at Sheffield, and F. R. S.*

"In July, 1720, a woman about 38 years of age was brought to me ; she had labored twelve years under an Epilepsy, which, from one fit a month, was come to four or five violent ones every day, each continuing an hour, or an hour and a half ; by which she was rendered mopish and silly, and incapable to take care of her house and family. Her husband was reduced in his circumstances from his affection and care for her, having got and followed all the advice he could. Evacuations of all kinds had been tried ; the epileptic and cephalic tribe of medicines had been ransacked, and many other medicines had been used in vain, the disease growing more severe. Her fit always began in her leg, toward the lower end of the *gastrocnemii* muscles, and in a moment reached her head, threw her down, foaming at the mouth, with terrible distortions of the mouth, neck and joints. Whilst I talked with her she fell down in a fit : I examined the leg, and found no swelling, hardness, laxness or redness different in that place from what was in the other leg : but suspecting from her fit beginning always at that part, that the cause of her disease lay there, I immediately plunged a scalpel about two inches into it, where I found a small indurated body, which I separated from the muscles, and then took it up with a forceps ; it proved a hard cartilaginous substance or ganglion, about the size of a very large pea, seated on a nerve, which I cut asunder, and took out the tumor. She instantly came out of the fit, cried out she was well, and never after had a fit, but recovered her former vigor both of body and mind."

From an attentive examination of numerous cases of this disease and of much that has been written respecting it, I am convinced that with many Epileptics there is a predisposition to this disease from an acquired or inherited greater sensibility or irritability, than other persons possess.

It is this peculiar condition of the whole nervous system that causes certain individuals to be affected by mental or corporeal impressions that produce little or no effect upon others. Every practitioner has seen cases apparently arising from dentition, from worms or other intestinal irritation, and I have just quoted a case where disease of a nerve appeared to cause it. Such affections produce Epilepsy however, in consequence of the very excitable condition of the brain and nervous system, already alluded to. Thus many cases of Epilepsy I apprehend, arise not from organic disease of the brain, but from such an excitable state of this organ, that any violent irritation in any part of the body transmitted to the brain will cause a rush of blood to it and produce an attack of Epilepsy. After repeated attacks and repeated congestions of blood in the brain, undoubtedly some organic changes will be found in this organ, but such changes are probably oftener effects than causes.

No doubt this excessive irritability or excitability of the brain and nervous system is hereditary. It may be acquired by the mother by a life of bodily indolence and mental excitement, and be transmitted to her offspring, or it may be acquired by the child without hereditary tendency by neglecting to exercise and develope all the powers of the body equally, and by constant excitement of the brain until it becomes the predominant organ and a nervous temperament produced.

Epilepsy is sometimes epidemic or contagious among females of feeble constitution and excitable nervous systems. Dr. Meyer of Bonn states that a girl at a school, attended both by boys and girls, was seized with Epilepsy, and soon after about twenty girls were similarly affected. Most of the girls were approaching the age of puberty and were of a highly excitable temperament. None of the boys were affected.

Prevention. — From what has been stated it is evident that preventive measures may be of great service.

These are obvious ; consisting in efforts calculated to develope and strengthen the corporeal powers and not to unduly excite the brain and nervous system.

With children and young persons who are strongly predisposed to this disease or exhibit a tendency to attacks of it, great care is necessary. Instead of seeking various amusements for them, and striving to excite their minds and exalt their sensibility, their minds should be permitted to run to waste, if I may so say, while the utmost pains should be taken to improve and strengthen the body by exercise in the open air.

Treatment. — It is obvious that this should vary with the cause. If Epilepsy arises from organic disease of the brain or skull there is little or no hope of recovery, unless it arises from a depressed bone or from some defect of the skull that an operation may remedy. If it arises from irritation in other parts of the system it may often be cured.

The physician then in attempting to cure Epilepsy should first examine and ascertain the condition of every part of the body, of every organ, and thus endeavor to find the source of irritation that causes the attack. The state of the stomach, bowels, liver, uterus, kidneys, &c., should be carefully examined.

In cases where there is but little or no hope of recovery, much benefit may be derived from a very cautious course of diet. I have known a diet, consisting of one kind of vegetable, cause an interval in the paroxysms of Epilepsy of three months, while the interval was not over two weeks on ordinary diet of animal and vegetable food.

In some instances, especially in children, it is necessary

to take away blood, not so much with a view of curing the disease, as to prevent disorganization of the brain, from the violence and frequency of the paroxysms. All Epileptics would do well to live by rule and abstemiously, avoiding all stimulating drinks and whatever is likely to excite the system. I have known some to be free from attacks while confined to a vegetable diet. Some cases seem to be kept up from habit, or from very slight irritation. Such are often benefitted by narcotics and tonics.

Stramonium has been found particularly beneficial, and so have the preparations of Zinc in large doses.* The nitrate of silver has appeared to cure in many instances. Some French writers have great confidence in it. It should be given in large doses and continued for a long time. Setons and Tartar emetic pustules along the spine have proved beneficial. Turpentine sometimes cures. I have known a case which seemed to depend on disordered bowels cured by it, for five years.

Mental emotions sometimes prove beneficial. Music has sometimes weakened, and at length subdued the paroxysm. Powerful mental impressions often prevent attacks. Hence probably the efficacy of the powder of human skulls† and of medicines presented with mystery and formality.

---

* I have used both these remedies with good effect in the following manner. Take of the seeds of Stramonium and of Myrrh equal parts, mix and make into two grain pills — of these one may be given, once in twelve and sometimes once in eight hours. The preparations of Zinc should be given in large doses. Take of Oxide of Zinc two drachms, Extract of Gentian two scruples, make into forty pills with a few drops of some essential oil. Give one of these the first day, two the second, three the third, and thus increase to twelve and fifteen in the twenty-four hours.

† I have been applied to for some within a few days.

On the whole the practice has been very empirical in Epilepsy. My own experience is in favor of a large seton in the pit of the neck, warm bathing, and a spare, vegetable diet. This course has lengthened the intervals of the attacks more than any other I have seen adopted.

The following is a singular case.*

CASE LIX.—" *The consequences of a Crown piece swallowed by an Epileptic man. Communicated to the College by Dr. Coyte, of Yarmouth, Norfolk. Read at the College, Nov.* 11, 1773. Mr. ———, aged about 46, has been from his infancy subject to Epileptic fits.

" On the 12th of March, 1771, he was attacked with a very strong fit ; and the people who happened to be present, recollecting the custom of his introducing a crown piece between his teeth, which he constantly carried about him, to prevent the tongue from being bit, as formerly had been the case whenever he had a return of these fits ; with eagerness to serve him, let it slip down his throat. The surgeon, (Mr. Arnold, of Lowestoff,) was from home at the time this accident happened, but at his return found Mr. ——— in violent agony, complaining of being choked, and of the impossibility of passing any thing into his stomach ; whenever he endeavored to swallow, he was greatly convulsed. and complained much of pain in both his ears, at which time the crown piece was so low in the œsophagus that it was impossible to get it back again: it remained only to pass it into the stomach, which with the concurrent advice of another surgeon, (Mr. Turner, of Yarmouth,) was accomplished : his throat was inflamed and very painful for a long time,

---

* Medical Transactions of the College of Physicians of London, Vol. iii. p. 30.

attended with the utmost difficulty in swallowing; his
health after this was much as usual, though his fits were
observed to be not so violent or frequent as before.

"Previous to an illness which he had lately, and on
which account I was consulted, he had occasion to be
employed in fixing wine in deep vaults, and sometimes
stood, as it were, upon his head, and complained soon
after of a weight at his stomach, attended with a sickness
and a bitter taste in his mouth: thus he had continued
for some days with a fever; and I found him on the 19th
of Sept. 1772, feverish, languid and very sick at times,
with a disagreeable bitter taste in his mouth; no emetic
having been ventured on to remove the cause of his present disorders, which appeared to me to be chiefly owing
to foulness in the stomach and primæ viæ; I ordered
pulv. rad. ipecac. gr. ij. and waited the operation; it
puked him presently, and brought away a large quantity of
viscid bilious matter, and, without giving him the least uneasiness, relieved him greatly. I left him, with directions
to Mr. Arnold, to repeat the Ipecac. gr. ij. pro re nata; it
was repeated three times that day, and several times the
day or two following; and his fever went off, and his
health was returning; when, on the 26th of November,
1772, in the morning, he was very sick, and vomited
several times, and in vomiting brought up the crown
piece without any pain, after it had lain in the stomach
from the 12th of March, 1771, to the 26th of November,
1772. Mr. now enjoys a perfect state of health, and has
had no return of the Epileptic fits since that time.

"Yarmouth, (Norfolk,) July 6, 1773.

"P. S. The crown piece appeared black, and somewhat corroded round one part of the edge and surface."

To what was the apparent cure owing? To the
silver, or to the irritation of the stomach produced by the
crown piece?

HYPOCHONDRIASIS.

This disease is characterized by some dyspeptic symptoms, such as flatulence, uneasiness in the stomach or abdomen, extreme lowness of spirits and apprehension of great danger, from supposed disease of some part of the body. The hypochondriac talks perpetually of his bad health. Though his appetite remains good and he looks healthy, he will say he has lost his appetite and is constantly losing flesh.

His countenance and manner show that he is sincere and that he is really apprehensive of the danger which he predicts. He is wholly engrossed with self—and constantly attentive to his own sensations.

I have known a father, in whom I could discover no disease, regardless of the sickness and approaching death of a child, constantly saying that his own case was more severe and alarming.

Though Hypochondriasis has been considered a distinct disease, it does not appear to me to be anything but a form of insanity, or monomania, combined with dyspepsia. A disease of the brain, functional most usually, together with disorder of some of the digestive organs.

Pathology. — In treating of the sympathetic nerve it was observed, that Prof. Lobstein believed that disease of this nerve was the cause of Hypochondriasis.

M. Lower Villermay and others, attribute it to a morbid state, an excess of organic sensibility in the nervous structure of some of the abdominal viscera, especially of the stomach.

M. Georget, very high authority, considers it a disease of the brain.

It is certain that this disease most frequently appears to arise from causes affecting the brain, such as moral affections of a painful nature — but on examination after death of those long hypochondriacal, very frequently no disease whatever has been found in the brain. That it is often a functional affection of the nervous system I think is evident. Its intermittent character, as frequently there are exemptions from it for years, shows that organic disease is not its cause. It has been cured by attacks of other disease, as intermittent fever.

From several cases which I have seen, and from those I have found in medical works, I am inclined to believe that it is a disease essentially of the nervous system and usually of the brain — a variety of mental alienation consisting often in hallucinations of sense, or of sensibility relative to some organ of the body.

Injury of the head sometimes causes it. Mr. C. aged about 30, a healthy and industrious man, was injured in the head by a board falling upon it. In a few weeks he appeared to have recovered from this injury, but complained of loss of strength — inability to walk — and that the sun when it shone on his head disturbed him very much. For several years he did not walk a step, but was almost daily placed in his wagon, with an umbrella which he continually carried over his head even when the sun did not shine. In this way he travelled much, transacted business and appeared in good health.

The sincerity of his belief that he could not walk was once proved. His house caught fire while no one but himself was in it. He was found by the neighbors seated in his chair, scorched by the fire and nearly suffocated by the smoke.

The following case also seems to indicate that the brain is the seat of this disease.

CASE LX. — Mr. T. aged 50, a highly intelligent and respectable gentleman, complained of painful erections of the penis. He was asked if he had taken Spanish flies, as they produced such symptoms. He said he had not; but after some months he became convinced that he had taken them in some cider, which had been given him by a female several months previous. On this he constantly dwelt and consulted many physicians to rid him of the effects of the Spanish flies. He was considered hypochondriacal, like men who are frequently so from fancied venereal disease, or fancied disease from mercury, which they have taken for the cure of it. He finally became deranged, idiotic, and died. It may tend to support some of the claims of Phrenology, that his manners changed very strangely as regarded females from the first attack of priapism. He became exceedingly attentive and polite to them, delighted to be in their company, and his conversation was mostly concerning them. Even when quite idiotic, if roused into conversation it would be in relation to women.

Mental shock alone causes it. A young man having heard a lecture from Esquirol, on the hereditary nature of insanity, called to mind that some of his ancestors had been insane. He immediately became sick and soon after committed suicide.

The disease appears to originate from a variety of bodily affections, which affections would not, I apprehend, produce it, was not the brain and nervous system in a morbid or super-excitable state. A little disease of any organ of the body may give rise to Hypochondriasis when the brain is in this morbid condition. Bad teeth, causing pain of the head, supposed to arise from organic disease of the brain, have produced this disease, which passed away after the diseased teeth were extracted. Disease of a single nerve has appeared to produce Hypochondriasis.

20*

The following is an interesting instance, from *Ollivier on Diseases of the Spinal Marrow.*

CASE LXI. — "A woman, 49 years of age who had previously enjoyed good health, began, in the year 1820, to feel strange pains through her body, originating in the left side of the chest, and caused, as she thought, by a small scirrhous tumour which was developed in the left mamma, but which was not painful on pressure. These pains increased in intensity, and deprived her of all enjoyment of life. She tried intoxication, but that rather aggravated than alleviated the evil. Still the tumour in the mamma remained stationary, and never became sensible to pressure. The unhappy woman was forever recounting the miseries she suffered ; and, at last, tired of existence, and wishing to deliver herself from the tortures she endured, she threw herself, on the 5th November, 1822, from a window in the fourth story of the house where she lodged. She was carried to the hospital, where our author saw her immediately, with the following symptoms : — Stupor, pallor of the face, great dyspnœa, pulse small and slow, skin cold, paralysis and insensibility of the trunk and lower extremities. There were various injuries, of different parts of the body, which we shall pass over. She died on the evening of the 8th November.

Dissection. — " In the head, the meninges were found thickened, but very little water in the ventricles. The body of the 10th dorsal vertebra was fractured transversely, but without the slightest displacement of the fractured portions. In the vertebral canal, opposite the fracture, there was an extravasation of fluid blood on the exterior surface of the dura mater. The medulla spinalis appeared of its natural color and consistence.

" In the thorax, the small scirrhous tumour was examined, but presented no trace of inflammation or disease around it. There were various fractures of the ribs; but the cause of the patient's long-continued sufferings was now brought into view. In the left side of the chest, and just above the arch of the aorta, was found a tumour of a pyriform shape, the size of a hen's egg, covered by, and adherent to, the pleura on one side, and on the other, it was in contact with one of the dorsal vertebræ. From the upper part of the tumour arose a white cord, the size of a goose-quill, which was traced into the foramen between the first and second dorsal vertebræ. On examining the spinal marrow, at this part, the filaments of the anterior and posterior roots of the first dorsal nerve were distinctly seen directing their course, as usual, to the foramen, for the formation of the first dorsal. This nerve, after issuing from the spine, gave off, as usual, a posterior branch. The anterior branch (after communicating with the great sympathetic, and giving rise to an ascending twig that passed on to unite with the seventh cervical) suddenly enlarged in volume, and proceeding about an inch from the point where it gave off the ascending twig, it terminated in the summit of the tumour. In this course, its colour was not altered — its neurilema was thickened, and it lost itself in, and became blended with, the tumour in question. This tumour was white and elastic, presenting some cartilaginous spots on its posterior surface. On slitting open the nerve which served as a peduncle, the neurilema of the nerve was found to expand itself and form a sheath, as it were, for the tumour. This last, when slit open, presented a pulpy surface, of a whitish colour, and appearing to be formed of concentric fibres, without a trace of vessel of any kind in its composition."

No doubt this woman was considered hypochrodrical, and probably many cases so denominated, are perpetua-

ted if not caused, by physical disease in some part of the
body, though I apprehend that generally the disease is
merely functional.

Men of well stored minds, those who devote themselves to study and take but little exercise are thought
to be most subject to it, though I have seen several instances among farmers and other laborers, all of whom
however were men given to reflection. Aristotle remarked that men of learning were most subject to this
disease. It has been termed the disorder of literary men.
A long list might be furnished of men illustrious for their
literary labors who were hypochondrical. Tasso, Pascal,
Zimmerman, Cowper, Dr. Johnson, Jean Jaques Rousseau are instances. The latter has thus vividly described
his sufferings.

"My health," says Rousseau, after he had gone into
the country with Madame de Warens, "did not improve
I was as pale as death, and meagre as a skeleton ; I had
dreadful pulsation of arteries : — to finish myself, having
read among other things a little physiology, I set to work
to study anatomy ; and passing in review the multitude
and the play of the parts which compose my machine, I
was in expectation of finding them all put out of order
twenty times a day. Far from being astonished at finding
myself dying, I was only astonished that I continued to
live ; and that I did not read a description of any malady
which I did not at once believe myself to have. I am sure,
if I had never been ill, this fatal study would have made
me so. Finding in every disease the symptoms of my own
I thought I had them every one ; and I acquired in addition one still more cruel of which I thought myself free,
the fantasy of curing myself. It is difficult to avoid this
when one takes to reading books of medicine. By dint
of exploring, reflecting, and comparing, I conceived that
the foundation of all my ailments was a polypus of the

heart, and even a physician seemed struck with this notion. I exercised all the powers of my mind to find out how to cure a polypus of the heart, being resolved to undertake this wonderful case. It had been said that M. Fizes, of Montpellier, had cured a polypus of that sort: nothing more was requisite to inspire me with the desire of going to consult M. Fizes. The hope of being cured revived my courage and my strength."

On his way to Montpellier he engaged in a flirtation with a certain Madame de Larnage, which, for a while at least, cured all his complaints. " So Madame de Larnage," he continues, " takes me under hand, and adieu poor Jean Jaques! or rather, adieu fever, vapours and the polypus! I forgot during my journey that I was a sick man."

No doubt Hypochrondriacal persons may be injured, as was Rousseau by reading medical books, and they should be advised not to peruse them, but not so in my opinion as regards those who are in health. According to my observation, those persons who have, by reading or otherwise, obtained some correct knowledge of anatomy, of diseases, and of medicines, are less disposed to hyprochondia than those who are quite ignorant on these subjects, and they are certainly less liable to be duped by quackery and made to believe they have disorder when it does not exist, and that certain medicines have miraculous powers and will cure every disease. The disease has, I believe, increased with civilization, ease and luxury. A predisposition is given to it by undue excitement of the brain and nervous system, by the developement of this part of the organization disproportionately to the rest of the body. When therefore the nervous system becomes thus charged as it were, with disease by over-excitement, the least disturbance of any other part of the fabric may serve to develope hypochondriasis.

It cannot, I think, always depend, as some suppose, on disease of the Great Sympathetic nerve — for this nerve appears to preside over the secretions, and must if diseased disturb digestion, generation, &c. But Hypochrondriacs frequently have good appetites. The worst case I ever knew, was that of a man who for several years remained in a recumbent posture, fully of the opinion that if raised up he should die ; yet he appeared to be in good health, had a good appetite, digested his food without difficulty, and had no loss of his generative powers.

The Treatment. — In the first place the hypochondriac should change his habits, so as to remove the causes of his disease.   He should quit his studies and ordinary pursuits and seek diversion and health by journeying — by daily riding and walking, even until fatigued.   Often engaging in some new and exciting business is useful. Many cases may be cured by the adoption of such measures, without the use of medicines.   Sometimes, however, local irritation may perpetuate the disease ; therefore every organ and every tissue of the body should be examined and the cause of the continuance of the disease, ascertained, and removed by appropriate remedies. Sometimes it is kept up by gastric or intestinal irritations produced by stimulants.   These should be withheld.   In other cases atony of the digestive organs seems to prolong the disease, and then tonics are useful.

It is not well to always regard Hypochrondrasis as an ideal disease, for often it arises from physical disorder. This disorder should be ascertained and removed, and then the general remedies alluded to for invigorating the body and diverting the mind will remove the hypochondia.

But on the other hand it is not well to unite in opinion

with hypochrondriacs and regard, or pretend to regard
the symptoms of which they complain, as indicating
alarming disease. It is best, I think, to tell them the
truth — that they probably have some disease, but that
most of it is imaginary. In cases of long standing I have
seen good result from compelling patients to exercise.
A person in an adjoining town confined himself to his
room for above six years, believing that he was unable
to walk out of doors — that it would kill him if compelled. I assisted in carrying him against his will, some
distance from his house, leaving him to walk back to it
of himself. He did so, and has since then gradually
recovered. Many other cases have come to my knowledge of long continued hypochondria cured in the same
manner. Before resorting however, to any compulsory
measures, the most careful examination should be made
to see if the disease is not kept up by some physical
disorder, that such measures would not be likely to remove.

In a subsequent chapter, on the *Effects of mental attention on bodily organs*, will be found remarks applicable
to some of the forms of Hypochondriasis.

HYSTERIA.

It is difficult, without writing a volume, to describe
this "protean disease." It is mostly confined to the
female sex, though not so absolutely as some writers suppose. I have seen a genuine case in a young man, and
other undoubted cases are reported by various writers.
Dr. Trotter observes, that at the time of a great
disturbance among the British sailors, many of them had
hysteria. Dr. Armstrong saw several cases of Hysteria
in men. Though regular attacks of this disease are not

common, and in truth are very unfrequent, in men, yet
certain symptoms usually denominated hysterical when
occurring in females, are not very uncommon in males.

For the most part hysteria occurs in young and middle
aged females, of delicate constitution, indolent habits, and
highly susceptible nerves. In such as are easily affected
by slight emotions of either pleasure or pain, and who
give way to the impulse of their feelings. An attack or
fit of hysteria is characterised by sighing, sobbing, laughing or weeping, with a feeling of stiffness and suffocation
about the throat, with some affection of the head, heart,
the respiratory or muscular system. Sometimes the
attacks are slight, consisting of alternate high and low
spirits, sighing, laughing and weeping. In other cases
there is violent pain of the head, great difficulty of
breathing, convulsions, loss of voice, hoarse dry cough,
and a sense of suffocation, with the feeling of a ball rising
up into the throat. There is often retention of urine followed by a copious flow.

The varieties of hysteria as described by writers are
very numerous ; similating a great number of other diseases as Croup, Apoplexy, Epilepsy, Paralysis, Tetanus,
Peritonitis, Diseases of the joints, as hip disease and
white swelling, Disease of the spine, and of the breast.
That such affections, purely nervous, though resembling
organic diseases, exist, I have had abundant unpleasant
experience ; unpleasant, because of the protracted nature of such cases and the difficulty of curing them. In
fact, there seems to be no symptoms resulting from
organic disease, but what are also manifested without
any appreciable organic lesion.

But why are all these nervous affections denominated
hysterical? Some of them are witnessed in those who
do not exhibit any other symptoms of hysteria. I have
at the present time, three cases of that peculiar spina'

affection, denominated by Sir B. Brodie, hysterical. Two of the three females thus affected, have never exhibited any other symptoms of hysteria. They have been cupped and leeched and had setons and issues along the spine, all without benefit. In fact, though many things seemed for a time to benefit them, I cannot say that any thing actually has. One having become *enceinte* appears to be rapidly recovering. Other cases I have seen recover, through the agency, I believe of the mind, or owing to a change of circumstances that powerfully affected the mind and changed the current of thought, creating new emotions. All these affections I believe, depend upon a faulty organization or disease, either functional or organic, of the brain. But we know so little of this organ, and the opportunities are so unfrequent for investigating the nature of these complaints by post mortem examination, that it is impossible to say how the brain is affected, or what portion of it. Some of the varieties of nervous disease, I shall allude to again in the section on the *Effects of mental attention on bodily organs.*

General Causes of Hysteria. — Hysteria is no doubt often hereditary, but it may also be acquired. It is often attended by positive disorder of some of the viscera, particularly by a costive state of the bowels. This is, I apprehend, a consequence, instead of a cause of the disease. A predisposition is given to it by a course of life that excites the nervous system and enervates the physical powers. Neglect of exercise in the open air, of bodily labor, with devotion to study — to reading, especially of works that kindle the imagination — much attention to music, late hours, hot rooms, and luxurious seats, tend to produce a susceptible and excitable state of the nervous system, that constitutes the first link in the chain of hys-

terical disorders. Females thus educated are susceptible
of strong emotions from the most trifling causes, and
experience great pleasure or pain from trivial amusements or petty annoyances. The nervous system is
thus kept perpetually in excitement, and is very easily
disordered. A little additional irritation from disorder
in some other part of the system, or mental emotion,
may so disturb it as to produce an attack of hysteria.

Pathology. — Morbid anatomy has thrown no positive
light upon this disease. It has shown however, that it
does not usually consist in organic lesion appreciable by
our senses.

Sir Benjamin C. Brodie, in his valuable *Lectures Illustrative of certain Local Nervous affections*, observes, "I
have in several instances examined the parts to which
hysterical pains had been referred ; and in one very
aggravated case of the kind I made a careful dissection of
all the nerves by which they were supplied, but I have
never been able to discover in them any thing different
from what belonged to their natural condition. But
every part of the body has its corresponding point in the
brain, and a greater number of them have their corresponding points in the spinal chord also. Does the examination of these organs lead to any more satisfactory
result ? The best proof that it does not do so, is furnished by the following circumstance ; although so many
die of other diseases, who have suffered from hysteria
also, and the opportunities of examining the bodies of
hysterical patients after death, are therefore sufficiently
numerous, yet the works of the best morbid anatomists
contain no observations whatever on the subject. I have
had the opportunity of instituting post mortem examinations in three cases, in which the hysterical affections
were of so aggravated a kind as to be directly or indi-

rectly, the cause of death; and you shall know the result. In one of them the patient labored under a very severe hysterical pain in the side, and was liable, among various other hysterical symptoms, to fits, in which she was scarcely conscious of her own actions. It must have been in one of these attacks that a great number of needles were introduced into one of her legs, which afterwards occasioned much inflammation and effusion of serum into the cellular texture. The patient died, and the body was most carefully examined, but no morbid appearances of any kind could be discovered in it, except what belonged to the œdematous state of the leg. Another case is one to which I have referred already, in which the patient having long labored under an hysterical retention of urine, the bladder was found enormously distended, of a black color, the mucous membrane and muscular tunic being at the same time much attenuated. This patient was an unmarried female twenty-nine years of age. Having been previously indisposed for a considerable time, she was supposed to have sprained her wrist in lifting a heavy sauce-pan. From this time she was never free from pain, in the situation of the outer part of the lower extremity of the radius. The pain extended up the fore-arm, and downwards on the side. In November, 1814, about a month after the occurrence of the accident, she was admitted into the hospital. At this time the most careful examination could detect no alteration in the appearance of the limb, but she complained of a constant and intense pain, which extended from the supposed seat of the injury downwards to the fingers, upwards to the shoulder, and again downwards to the spine and sternum. She had great oppression and difficulty of respiration, occasional twitches of the muscles of the face, and any sudden motion of the hand aggravated all these symptoms, and then threw her into a state approaching to that of syncope; in which she was almost unconscious of all that happened, lying with her eyes wide open, and at last recovering with an hysterical sobbing. Her pulse was feeble, beating 120 times in a minute. Forty ounces of urine were drawn off from the bladder, but without any relief as to the other symptoms. The tongue became black and dry; the pulse more feeble; the belly tympanitic; the alvine evacuations being of a dark color. Then there was hiccough and vomiting: she became weaker and weaker, and died after the lapse of fourteen days from the time of her admission into the hospital. After death the brain and the thoracic and abdominal viscera were very carefully examined, but no morbid appearances were discovered in any one of them, with the exception of the peculiar condition of the bladder, which was described formerly, and two ulcers of the mucous membrane of the ileum, each not more than half an inch in length, but occupying almost the entire circumference of the intestine.

The female, who was the subject of the third case had labored under a paralytic affection of the lower limbs (*paraplegia*), which Dr. Seymour believed, with good reason, to be connected with, and the consequence of, hysteria. A practitioner whom she consulted, however, thought it advisable to have recourse to repeated bloodletting and other methods of depletion. The result was, the formation of extensive sloughs of the nates and of the soft parts covering the ankles. The patient was now admitted into the hospital, in a state of great exhaustion, and soon afterwards died. The brain and spinal chord were most carefully examined, in the presence of many of you who are now present, but it could not be discovered that they differed, in the smallest degree, from their natural condition; nor were there any signs of disease in the thoracic or abdominal viscera."

Some have placed the seat of this disease in the uterus. This is the most ancient opinion, and is embraced by some of the most distinguished of the moderns, though as it appears to me, on very insufficient evidence. The opinions of the ancients on this subject were founded upon extreme ignorance, or rather upon an entire mistake as to the situation of the uterus. This is evident by the following quotation. "The uterus," says Aretæus, "greatly resembles an animal. It moves itself to various parts of the body, sometimes upwards to the throat, then to the sides, oppressing the lungs, the heart, the diaphragm, the liver, and the intestines. It is an animal within an animal, and is constantly wandering. It loves good odors and approaches them, but dislikes bad odors and flies from them." Their practice conformed to their theory, thus they applied pleasant perfumes to the pubes, and assafoetida &c. to the throat.

They also equalled any of the moderns in attributing innumerable evils to the womb. Democritus in writing to Hippocrates says that *the womb is the origin of six hundred evils and innumerable calamities.*

Sydenham attributed hysteria to an "irregular flow of the animal spirits," but the majority of writers on this disease, have, I believe, considered uterine disturbance as its cause. Mr. Tate says that, "all the varieties of hysteria have one common cause, which is essential to its appearance ; namely, an irregular or defective menstruation."

Some place the seat of it, rather vaguely, in the nervous system, while others as M. Georget, consider it a disorder of the brain. I am inclined to believe this opinion correct. The most inveterate case of hysteria I have ever witnessed was that of a young lady who was free from the disease until after a severe injury of her head by a fall. Her mother and sisters were never hysterical.

21*

What physician but often sees disease of the uterus without any hysterical symptoms. We also see very hysterical females go through gestation and delivery as safely and in the same manner as females who are not subject to the disease. These facts daily noticed by physicians, seem to be wholly irreconcilable with the idea, that disorder of the uterus is the cause of hysteria.

Its exciting causes confirm me in the belief that the brain is the seat of the disease. Excitement of the feelings, disturbance of the affections, and a great variety of mental emotions produce an attack.

The sight of a person in a paroxysm of hysteria sometimes causes another to be similarly affected. In the Northern States it is very common in the winter for the young people of both sexes to assemble in large numbers for sleigh-riding. On one such occasion, when a large party had stopped at a public house and partaken of wine and other refreshments, a young lady was attacked with hysteria, and soon a majority of the females present were similarly affected.

But why are females more liable to hysterical complaints than men? Because they have from nature a more delicate and susceptible brain and nervous system, a nervous system which I apprehend is not only more excitable, but endowed with sensibilities to which men are strangers. It is owing to this, to a difference in the brain and nervous system that gives to the female a greater intensity of emotions, more variable desires, quicker apprehension, and a more kindling imagination. The duties of a mother are so peculiar, requiring patient, long-enduring self-immolation in the discharge of them, that a nervous system different from that of man as to instincts and sensations is requisite. This delicate and susceptible nervous system of the female is easily disordered, especially by mental emotions. Hence anger, terror, grief, jealousy, remorse, unfortunate love and prostrated hopes, by disordering this system produce hysteria. The same emotions also derange the uterine functions not unfrequently. So strong impressions on the organs of sense, irritation of the alimentary canal, &c., may produce an hysterical paroxysm in a female by arousing into morbid action her very excitable nervous system.

Prevention. — Methods of prevention are obvious, consisting in attention to the physical education of girls. On this subject I would say to parents, using for the most part the language of another, — Let your first care be to give your little girls a good *physical* education. Let their early years be passed, if possible, in the country, gathering flowers in the fields, and partaking of all the free exercises in which they delight. When they grow older do not condemn them to sit eight listless hours a day over their books, their work, their maps, and their music. Half the number of hours, will in every respect, both as to mental and bodily improvement be the better for them. Let them partake of every active exercise not absolutely unfeminine. Let them rise early, and retire early to rest. Let them ride, walk, run, dance, in the open air. Encourage the merry and innocent diversions in which the young delight ; let them under proper guidance, explore every hill and valley; let them plant and cultivate the garden, and make hay when the summer sun shines, and surmount all dread of a shower of rain or of boisterous wind; and above all, let them take no *medicine, cordials, essences,* except when the physician orders them. The demons of hysteria and melancholy might hover over a group of young ladies so brought up; but they would not find one of them upon whom they could exercise their power. Such advice,

to the parents and guardians of young girls, I deem it the
duty of physicians to give, and to strongly remonstrate
against the adoption of a different course.

Treatment. — No disease is deserving of more careful
study than hysteria, as some of its varieties similate other
diseases of a grave character, and without careful investigation, very erroneous practice may be adopted. The
exciting cause should be sought for and removed. This
often consists of intestinal or uterine derangement, which
should be remedied, and then the whole system should
be strengthened by tonics and exercise.

During an attack the treatment should vary according
to its intensity and exciting cause. Sometimes it is necessary to bleed freely to prevent sanguineous congestion in
the head. This is very proper treatment in young
females who are atacked by hysteria in consequence of
the suppression of the catamenial discharge. Emetics
are indicated if there are symptoms of gastric irritation
such as retching and pain of the stomach. Stimulating
enema particularly of turpentine, are often beneficial,
and in all cases, a torpid state of the bowels should be
avoided. When mental emotions cause the attack, laudanum and sulphuric ether will usually relieve. Asafœt-
ida, musk, castor, and valerian are also useful.

After the removal of the local irritation and the system remains in an irritable and feeble state, then tonics,
particularly the preparations of iron, nourishing diet,
gentle exercise in the open air, pleasing occupations
and agreeable society are useful. It should however
ever be borne in mind that hysteria and many nervous
diseases are increased by notice, and neglect is often the
best remedy. Sometimes the return of a paroxysm is
prevented by the fear of the remedy that is to be resorted
to. Dr. Armstrong cured a young lady, or prevented a

recurrance of a paroxysm, by ordering her feet to be burned by a hot poker whenever a fit occurred.

TETANUS.

This alarming disease consists in violent spasms of the voluntary muscles while the mind remains unaffected. It has long been divided into idiopathic and traumatic — idiopathic when it arises from various general causes, as from cold, from sleeping in the open air, and from narcotic poisons. It also occurs in the course of other diseases, as in the latter stages of fever. It is called traumatic when it arises from injuries, wounds, burns, &c. M. Hall, divides the disease into central and centripetal, the former, produced by disease within the spinal canal, the latter by wounds, or other injuries.

I refer the reader to other works on Tetanus, particularly to that of Curling, for a full detail of the symptoms and progress of this disease, though I wish to remark here what has not been noticed by many writers on Tetanus, that in some cases the most violent spasms produce no pain whatever.

The following is a recent case of the kind.

CASE LX. — Edmund Avery, aged 18, while assisting in repairing a house, August 22nd., had one of his legs crushed by the falling of a part of the building. The tibia and fibula of his left leg, were fractured about midway between the ankle and knee. The bones at the place of fracture did not protrude, but there was a severe lacerated wound above the outer ankle which exposed the fibula, and another severe wound below the ankle. Sixty drops of laudanum were administered and after the limb was dressed he had but little pain and no spasms during the night. The next day the pulse being full he was bled eighteen ounces. The fifth day the wounds began to discharge and appeared to be doing very well. He continued to improve, complained of but little pain, and had no spasms until the 2nd of September, eleven days after the injury. On the morning of that day, after dressing the wound, which discharged freely, and appeared to be healing, he observed that he had taken cold he thought, as he had some soreness and stiffness of the throat. Tetanus was immediately suspected, though no symptoms were observed indicating any change or danger, excepting slight stiffness and soreness of the throat, which the patient attributed to a cold.

Sixty drops of laudanum were administered, and soon after 100 drops by enema. Cupping along the spine was resorted to and blisters applied. The next day he was not able to open his jaws more than half an inch, the pulse was rapid, he was in profuse perspiration and complained of pain at the sternum. Spasms had become frequent, the diseased limb was drawn up and distorted; the other limbs and the muscles of his back were also affected by spasms, but throughout the whole of them he declared they were not painful, and just before he expired observed that he should recover if he could get the phlegm from his throat. Opium and calomel were freely administered so long as he was able to swallow, and laudanum was given in enemas. He expired on the fourth day after the first appearance of the Tetanic symptoms. I consider this case unusual from the absence of pain, and from the healthy apperance and free discharge of the wound even until his death. I examined the leg and the wounds very carefully, but could find nothing unusual or that appeared to have given rise to the disease. The muscles, ligaments and nerves were not inflamed, but on the contrary appeared rather more full and flaccid than natural.

I witnessed a fatal case of Hydrophobia a few years since in this city, and the symptoms very closely resembled those of the case described. The case of hydrophobia was caused by a wound in the back of the hand from the teeth of a dog. The symptoms of hydrophobia appeared in about two weeks, and the person died in three days. He was able to swallow, though not without extreme difficulty, and not without slight convulsions. Avery, swallowed also with difficulty even the mildest liquids and those at all irritating he could not. The same dog, immediately after having bitten the person alluded to, bit another in the thigh, producing a large ragged wound which however healed kindly and the gentleman has since enjoyed good health. The dog was killed soon after having thus attacked these individuals, but the same day he had bitten two other dogs, both of which afterwards sickened and died of hydrophobia. The symptoms they manifested were quite different. One ate and drank well throughout his sickness, though he had paroxysms of violent mania and convulsions, in one of which he died. When the paroxysms ceased, he appeared well and his eyes natural. I examined his stomach, throat and brain. There was no inflammation in either or other marks of disease : but the stomach was crowded and distended with rags, wool, grass, straw, and balls of the hard manure of other animals.

The other dog would not swallow and seemed perpetually mad and disposed to bite. He appeared to be in constant agony. His eyes were blood-shot. On examining his body after death, the mucous membrane of the fauces and glottis was found inflamed, the brain and its membranes highly injected with blood, and there was some effusion of serum into the ventricles and between the membranes. His stomach was natural. I regret that I was not able to examine the spinal marrow in any of the cases to which I have referred. This is about all I know of hydrophobia from personal observation. The only case I have ever witnessed, had I not known to have arisen from the bite of a dog supposed to be mad, I should have called a case of Tetanus, and not an uncommon one.

Pathology. — Inflammation of the spinal marrow, or its membranes are supposed by many of the most distinguished pathologists, to give rise to tetanus. Certain it is, that inflammation of one or both of these structures has been observed after tetanus in numerous cases. Baron Larrey states that in the numerous inspections of the bodies of the soldiers who died of tetanus in the hospitals of Louvain after the battle of Waterloo, he continually noticed traces of inflammation in the spinal cord, with serous effusion more or less of a reddish color within the sheath. Armstrong mentions a case produced by the odontoid process pressing on the spinal cord. In a case in the Massachusetts hospital there was softening of the spinal cord.

Billard (Treatise on the Diseases of Infants,) says, he has seen but two cases of this disease in young infants, and that "on dissection he found nothing more than an effusion of a quantity of coagulated blood in the spine. The blood was effused between the two laminæ of the tunica arachnoidea, and filled the whole of the medullary canal from the medulla oblongata to the sacral region."

In the London Medical Gazette, for 1838, is a case in which only one half of the body was affected by tetanus. Extreme soreness of the skin was the first symptom of disease. It was cured by leeches over the spine.

Numerous other instances might be referred to, showing

that disease of the spinal cord is very frequently found after death from tetanus, and this view of the disease ought to have much influence in its treatment. Curling, thinks tetanus consists in a peculiar morbid action in the tractus motorius, the intimate nature of which is altogether beyond our comprehension.

In some cases no inflammation or other disease of the spinal cord has been observed after careful examination; and again the spinal cord has been found inflamed without symptoms of tetanus. It appears to me, however, that the disease is always dependent upon irritation, if not actual organic disease of the medulla spinalis, and is well explained by M. Hall's theory of the independent functions of this organ.

Treatment. — When Tetanus arises from the partial division of nerves, the complete division of them will sometimes immediately arrest the disease. I have seen this in one case relieve the most violent spasms. But in such cases the disease is not fully established; when it is, it is seldom cured.

General bleeding is rarely necessary. I have in several cases seen it resorted to, but never with benefit, and I have known Tetanus occur after injuries accompanied by profuse hemorrhage. Tonics and stimulants have sometimes proved beneficial. Dr. Hosack cured several cases of traumatic Tetanus by the liberal use of wine. In one case he administered three gallons in the course of three days, and the patient recovered. In all his cases the tetanic symptoms appeared immediately or shortly after the injury. General Moreau informed Dr. Hosack, that lock-jaw was of rare occurrence in an army when they first took the field, but that it was produced by the slightest wounds when the soldiers had become

22

fatigued and debilitated by long marches and frequent battles.

The treatment should vary with the exciting cause, state of the pulse, duration of the disease, &c. I should commence the treatment by giving croton oil to move the bowels, and if the pulse was not feeble, should apply leeches and cups along the spine, then blisters or the actual cautery, to the spinal region, and administer opium freely by the mouth, and by enemas. If debility and feebleness of pulse I should give wine. In some cases, amputation of the wounded limb has saved the patient, but generally it has proved unsuccessful. The same may be said of mercury. Colchicum I should think might be serviceable. In India they seem to have been quite successful in curing traumatic Tetanus. An anonymous writer in the London Medical Repository, vol ix, p. 300, says, " It is pretty generally known, that in the symptomatic Tetanus from wounds which occur in the East Indies, about one in four recover; and the usual practice which is followed there, is the use of mercury, both internally and locally, with the exhibition of large quantities of opium, spirits, or wine. Some have found the warm bath useful ; and in the hands of others, the effusion of water of the temperature of the surrounding atmosphere (which is about 80 deg. of Fahrenheit) has proved a powerful auxiliary in the treatment of the disease. It generally proves fatal before the seventh day. At first, the spasmodic affection is generally confined to the parts immediately above the wound ; but the whole side of the body is soon afterwards thrown into violent spasmodic contractions ; and if a tournaquet or tight ligature is placed above the wounded part, so as to compress the nerves, the spasms will be relieved, and very generally prevented recurring. This measure is frequently of great use in enabling the patient to take a little sustenance, or to swallow his medicine."

CHOREA — ST. VITUS'S DANCE.*

This disease is characterised by irregular twitchings and involuntary contractions of various muscles of the body. It is a kind of *muscular insanity*, by which the limbs are irresistibly moved in various directions.

It is often preceded by dyspeptic symptoms, pain of the stomach, flatulence, constipation, and tumid bowels. Sometimes vertigo, slight tremors, and illusions of sight occur, before the movements of the muscles are noticed.

---

* " Chorus Sancti Viti, or St. Vitus's dance ; the lascivious dance Paracelsus calls it, because they that are taken with it, can do nothing but dance till they be dead, or cured. It is so called for that the parties so troubled were wont to go to St. Vitus's Chapels for help ; and, after they had danced there awhile, they were certainly freed. 'Tis strange to hear how long they will dance, and in what manner, over stools, forms, tables ; even great bellied women sometimes (and yet never hurt their children) wil. dance so long that they can stir neither hand nor foot, but seem to be quite dead. One in red clothes they cannot abide. Music above all they love ; and therefore magistrates in Germany will hire musicians to play to them, and some lusty, sturdy companions to dance with them. This disease hath been very common in Germany, as appears by those relations of Schenkius, and Paracelsus in his book of madness, who brags how many several persons he hath cured of it. Felix Platerus (*de Mentis Alienat. cap.* 3.) reports of a woman in Basle whom he saw. that danced a whole month together. The Arabians call it a kind of *palsie*. Bodine, in his fifth book, *de* Repub. cap. 1., speaks of this infirmity ; Monavius, in his last epistle to Scoltizius, and in another to Dudithus, where you may read more of it." — *Burton's Anatomy of Melancholy*, Vol. 1.

"He, St. Vitus, was a Sicilian youth who, together with Modestus and Crescentia, suffered martyrdom at the time of the persecution of the christians, under Diocletian, in the year 303. The Legends respecting

In some cases the convulsive action of the muscles is slight, and confined to the face or to one side of the body, but not unfrequently they increase to such a degree as to prevent patients from walking, and from dressing or feeding themselves. A slight derangement or feebleness of the intellectual faculties is often noticed. It is usually unattended by fever, and in many cases no complaint is made of pain. In some cases there is pain of the head. It is sometimes connected with Epilepsy and Insanity, and sometimes terminates in these diseases. It bears a great resemblance to Hysteria and Epilepsy. The disease is mostly confined to youth, and to those between the ages of eight and twenty, and who are of a nervous temperament.

---

him are obscure, and he would certainly have been passed over without notice among the innumerable apocryphal martyrs of the first centuries, had not the transfer of his body to St. Denys, and thence, in the year 836, to Corvey, raised him to a higher rank. From this time forth, it may be supposed that many miracles were manifested at his new sepulchre, which were of essential service in confirming the Roman faith among the Germans, and St. Vitus was ranked among the fourteen saintly helpers (Nothhelfer or Apotheker). His altars were multiplied, and the people had recourse to them in all kinds of distresses, and revered him as a powerful intercessor. As the worship of these saints was however at that time stripped of all historical connections, which were purposely obliterated by the priesthood, a legend was invented at the beginning of the fifteenth century, or perhaps even so early as the fourteenth, that St. Vitus had, just before he bent his neck to the sword, prayed to God that he might protect from the dancing mania all those who should solemnize the day of his commemoration, and fast upon its eve, and that thereupon a voice from heaven was heard, saying, "Vitus, thy prayer is accepted." Thus St. Vitus became the patron saint of those afflicted with the dancing plague, as St. Martin, of Tours, was at one time the succourer of persons in small-pox; St. Antonius of 'those suffering under the hellish fire,' and as St. Margaret was the Juno Lucina of puerperal women." — *Hecker's Epidemics of the middle ages.*

Causes. — The opinion of Dr. Hamilton that Chorea usually arises from the irritation of feculent matter in the bowels is generally considered incorrect. It is said worms have produced it, and no doubt it does sometimes arise from intestinal irritation. It has been caused by falls on the head, and wounds penetrating the brain, also by fright, jealousy, anger, and other strong mental emotions.

Females and youth, and those of a nervous temperament are most subject to this disease. It is also hereditary. Repelled cutaneous eruptions, and the suppression of habitual discharges sometimes excites this disease. Dentition and parturition occasionally cause it, also onanism, and the retention or suppression of the menses. Sometimes it arises from the extension of other diseases of the nervous system, as epilepsy, hysteria, and mental alienation.

Pathology. — Few die of this disease, hence but little light has been thrown upon it, by post mortem examinations.

When we notice the most characteristic symptoms of Chorea, are, inability to combine and regulate the motions essential to walking, standing, &c., and then call to mind that the researches of Rolando, Flourens, Bouillaud and Magendie, show that this power belongs to the cerebellum, we shall be lead to consider this organ the seat of the disease. I am disposed to believe this view of Chorea to be correct, though, no doubt, other portions of the nervous system, the cerebrum, the medulla oblongata and medulla spinalis are sometimes implicated, though I apprehend in such instances Chorea would not result, unless the functions of the cerebellum were disturbed.

Serres found in one case the tubercula quadrigemina inflamed. Dr. Armstrong alludes to a case in

22*

which increased vascularity of the spinal cord was observed. Not unfrequently the region of the cerebellum is the seat of pain, especially during the greatest violence of the disease. Boutelle refers to such instances. The same author states that he has known the disease to arise from falls on the head. The occipital region has been found hotter than natural in Chorea. In the 15th volume of the Lancet is a case of a girl who menstruated a little at six years of age, and fully when eight. The mammæ were also developed at this age. This girl had no power to control the action of the voluntary muscles, and on examination the occipital region over the cerebellum was found to be very perceptibly hotter than natural. Other methods of treatment having proved unavailing, she was leeched over the cerebellar region, and had cold water applied to that part.

This course arrested the spasmodic action of the muscles and stopped the menses for eight months, when both returned, and were again cured by the same means.

In support of the opinion that the cerebellum is the seat of Chorea, it should be recollected that the disease occurs about the time of puberty, when there is supposed to be increased activity and rapid enlargement of this organ.

In the 25th volume of the Medico Chirurgical Review, is an account of a fatal case of Chorea, in which, on careful examination of every part of the system but the spine, nothing unusual was discovered, except two small spicula of bone, one from the orbital plate of the frontal bone, the other from the sphenoid, a quarter of an inch in length.

Dr. Stiebel, a late German writer on Chorea, who has had much experience in this disease, believes it arises from an irritation of the motor nerves of the spinal marrow, or of the medulla oblongata, depending on inflammation or turgescence. He has usually found, some one of the vertebræ painful.

Treatment. If there is pain of the head, or if it is unnaturally hot, or if there is tenderness or pain of any part of the spine, leeches and blisters should be applied to the back of the neck and along the spine. I usually apply blisters to the back of the neck, even if there is no pain of the head, and believe I have seen much benefit result from this practice. If disorder of the bowels or menstrual disturbance, the usual remedies for such complaints should be had recourse to, and then tonics and narcotics will usually effect a cure. The preparations of iron, especially the carbonate, are useful. Arsenic has sometimes arrested the disease after the failure of other remedies. Showering with cold water, or plunging the patient for an instant in cold water, has proved beneficial. This practice is recommended by Dupuytren.

Antispasmodic and narcotic medicines are often necessary. Conium, stramonium, and morphine, particularly the latter, I have known highly serviceable.

As mental emotion aggravates the disease, the utmost pains should be taken to preserve a quiet and cheerful state of mind. Nothing should be said to those afflicted with this disease respecting their involuntary motions, and their attention should be directed from them, as much as possible. Chorea uncomplicated with other disease, I believe, never proves fatal.

Dr. Stiebel's course of treatment consists in leeches and blisters along the spine, and calomel given as a derivative. If not soon relieved by this course, he showers the back with cold water. He states that the disease is generally cured by this treatment between the fourteenth and twenty-first day, but should not this happen

it may be left to nature, which almost always perfects
the cure. The preparations of iron he has sometimes
found useful, but he appears to believe that many inert
and useless medicines have acquired a reputation in the
treatment of Chorea, merely from having been administered, at the time, nature was affecting a cure.

DELIRIUM TREMENS.

It is very singular, that this, now common disease, was
almost wholly overlooked or not known as a distinct disease, until within the last forty years. Unquestionably it
is now vastly more frequent than in former times, still it
is not probable, that no cases occured before the time
mentioned. They were confounded with phrenzy.

The January number of the Medico Chirurgical Review, for 1839, contains three cases of this disease, taken
from the works of Stoll. These cases occurred in 1773,
and are detailed by him in a Chapter on the Causes and
Seat of *Phrenzy.*

The first account of this disease, that attracted the
notice of the profession, was published in a small tract,
by Samuel Burton Pearson, M. D. As it is brief, valuable and rare, I insert it here.

" *Observations on Brain Fever. By Samuel Burton
Pearson, M. D.*

" *Brain Fever.* — At the earnest solicitation of several
people who have been afflicted with this grievous malady, 1 offer this small treatise to the public. Multifarious
and repugnant theories on the science of life still continue
to agitate the medical world. Galen's writings, after
the extinction of literature for several ages, were again
revived, and produced innumerable controversies. The

accrimonious opposition of the Galenists and Arabians, and the complete overthrow of the latter, are well known to every reader. The chemists attacked the Galenists with fury, and they sustained a defeat. Different sects have originated from Stahl, Hoffman, Boerhaave, Cullen, and Brown. A medical review will convince any one how the faculty worry each other at the present day, about their different dogmas, with much injury to themselves and patients. For the above reasons I disavow all theory, and briefly state the circumstances as they occurred to me at the patient's bed side. Out of ninety-three cases that have been treated by the principles here adopted, not one has fallen a victim to the disorder; but, when a contrary mode has been attempted, few have recovered, and those only whose constitutions were sufficiently vigorous to resist its ravages.

" I have called it Brain Fever, because it is universally known in Newcastle and its vicinity by that term. The same observation extends to putrid fever.

Cause. — Frequent and excessive intoxication.

Description. — It is preceded by tremors of the hands; restlessness; irregularity of thought; deficiency of memory; anxiety to be in company; dreadful nocturnal dreams, when the quantity of liquor through the day has been insufficient; much diminution of appetite, especially an aversion to animal food; violent vomiting in the morning; and excessive perspiration from trivial causes. The above symptoms increase; the pulse becomes small and rapid, the skin hot and dry; but soon a clammy sweat bedews the whole surface of the body; confusion of thought arises to such a height, that objects are seen of the most hideous forms, and in positions that it is physically impossible they can be situated; the patient generally sees flies or other insects, or pieces of money, which he anxiously desires to possess; and often occupies much time in conversations of negotiation, if he be a commercial man. Often, for many days and nights, he will continue without rest, notwithstanding every effort is made on the part of the physician to appease his mind by variety of conversation, and variety of stimuli. He frequently jumps suddenly out of bed in pursuit of a phantom, and holds the most ineffable contempt for the practitioner, if he do not concur in his proceedings. He commonly retains the most pertinacious opinion that he is not in his own house, and that some of his dearest relations have sustained a serious injury. During the concourse of these symptoms, he often can answer medical questions properly for a short space of time, and then relapses into the raving state.

Distinction. — It is distinguished from putrid fever, in never being contagious, or having purple spots; or ever having a cadaverous smell; or ever being received from human effluvia; and in the delirium being much more impetuous. It is distinguished from inflammation of the brain and its membranes, by not having so vehement a fever; or redness and turgescense of the eye and face; or impatience of light or noise; or hard pulse; and by opposite causes, and opposite method of cure.

Method of Cure. — A full dose of opium should be immediately administered in a glass of wine, and repeated in smaller doses for several hours successively; the quantity of which should be regulated by the constitution of the patient, habit of intoxication, degree of the disease, and other concomitant circumstances. The patient, if he eagerly request it, may be allowed to walk from room to room, and the most consoling language should be used by his attendants. The debility of the system should be resisted by sherry gruel, cold wine, and porter and soup; which may be given in sufficient quantity, as the stomach, in this complaint, is very tenacious of what it receives. I never saw the bark, blistering, or effusion of cold water on the head, of any use. Every unnecessary restraint should be carefully avoided ; therefore the strait-jacket, which is so universally employed, is the most injurious remedy that can be applied ; for, by the perpetual efforts the patient uses to rid himself from confinement, he excites profuse sweating, debilitates the muscular fibre, and soon exhausts the vital principle. If the above mode of treatment be successful, or at least affords the unhappy sufferer a chance of recovery ; the impoverishing the system by bleeding, strait-jacket, or abstinence from invigorating remedies and diet, must be extremely mischievous.

Newcastle upon Tyne, July, 1801."

This tract had but a limited circulation, confined chiefly to the friends and acquaintance of Dr. Pearson. He called it Brain Fever as it was generally known by that name in his neighborhood. Twelve years after this, in 1813, Dr. Armstrong, published in the Edinburgh Medical and Surgical Journal, two articles upon this disease, which he denominated Brain Fever from *intoxication*. He refers to the small tract of Dr. Pearson, and says, to that "he was first indebted for any thing like an accurate description of the disease."

The same year Dr. Thomas Sutton, of London, published "Tracts" on the same disease, which he denominate l "Delirium Tremens."

It is qu.te evident from the perusal of these early publications on this disease, that it was well known at that time to the medical profession, but had not been described, as a distinct disease, or a disease arising from the use of intoxicating liquor.

The *symptoms* are well described by Dr. Pearson, also its cause, "frequent and excessive intoxication." But, the long and habitual use of alcoholic liquors, without causing what is called intoxication, will produce it. I have seen several such cases. I have known individuals who exhibited the symptoms of Delirium Tremens, and on inquiry of some of their friends and associates, have been surprised to find them ignorant of the fact, that the individuals affected, made use of alcoholic drink. On further inquiry, however, of servants, grocers or nearest relatives, I ascertained they had, for a considerable time, used such liquors, but not so as to produce intoxication.

It has been said that the use of opium, and other narcotics causes delirium tremens ; but this disease arises so very rarely from any other cause than the use of intoxicating liquor, that this may, with propriety, be considered almost the sole cause. I have never seen a case produced by any thing else, but a medical friend has assured me, that he once saw a genuine case from the use of opium.   He was not certain, however, but the patient was in the habit of washing down the opium, with a little alcoholic drink.   The disease sometimes, though rarely, arises from the use of only a small quantity of intoxicating liquor   Dr. Sutton relates the case of a lady who had the delirium tremens, in consequence of the daily use of the Tincture of Lavender.

According to my observation, the disease seldom attacks a person while in the use of intoxicating drink. It supervenes usually, after some slight illness, that has caused the relinquishment of the accustomed stimulus. A slight attack of pneumonia often precedes the delirium. The latter comes on after the patient is convalescent from the affection of the lungs.

Sometimes, however, the disease appears to be the immediate consequence of intoxication.   Individuals have gone to sleep deeply intoxicated, and waked up

with delirium tremens. I have seen two cases that occurred without any relinquishment of spirituous liquor.
Such cases I believe, are in some respects different from
those that occur after the usual stimulus has been withheld for several days. They yield less readily to opiates,
and bear depletion better. Some even require bleeding.
One of the patients thus attacked, was much benefitted
by bleeding.

Mental shock, has, I believe, considerable agency in
causing this disease.

A man was arrested for the crime of theft. He appeared at the trial to be in good health, until his daughter,
the only positive evidence of his guilt, testified against
him. Instantly his countenance changed, he trembled
excessively, soon became delirious, and manifested the
usual symptoms of delirium tremens for thirty-six hours,
when he died. He was not considered an intemperate
man, and was never known to be intoxicated, though he
made use of spirituous liquor.

I think the disease is sometimes caused by apprehension
of it. A person who uses intoxicating drink to excess
becomes fearful of an attack of delirium tremens, when-,
ever he is affected with any disorder of the system.
This fear prevents sleep. In this way, I am confident, I
have seen two cases occur.

Pathology. — I have examined with great care the
bodies of five men who died of delirium tremens. In
all these cases there was effusion of serum between the
membranes of the brain, and the tunica arachnoidea was
highly injected. This was more particularly true about
the decussation of the optic nerves, and also in the cerebellum. The cerebellum in three cases seemed to be
harder than natural and the corpus dentatum unusually

23

soft and partially disorganized. Neither case exhibited disease of the stomach.

Treatment. — From the success which attended the practice of Dr. Pearson, already quoted, it is evident that the course recommended by him is not a bad one. I have always relied upon opium, and have been so generally successful, that I cannot with propriety recommend any other course. I have however uniformly avoided a costive state of the bowels and often combined calomel with the opium.

I usually commence the treatment with small doses of calomel with two or three grains of opium given every two hours. If this does not produce sleep after four or five doses have been taken, I generally move the bowels, and then repeat the opium. I have given half an ounce of laudanum at a dose and with apparent benefit.

The worst cases have been cured solely by opium. There may however be cases where opium would be useless or improper, and depletion necessary. I deemed bleeding necessary in one case, that of a young man of full habit and strong pulse, and in whom the disease occurred without any abandonment of intoxicating drink. The bleeding mitigated the violence of the delirium, but did not entirely overcome it. Opium however did. The bleeding I deemed necessary to prevent apoplexy or disorganization of the brain.

I have in several cases administered emetics, and seen them given by others, but have never witnessed much if any benefit from them. I have recently seen a case prove fatal in which emetics had been given.

A long walk appears to benefit some patients. A man in this town broke from his keepers in the night and wandered about the town for several hours — the next morning he was tranquil, slept and recovered. A medical friend has cured by inducing strangury. I have seen one case that recovered without the use of any medicine. The patient for the most part was suffered to walk about accompanied by attendants. After three days of excitement, talking and travelling, he went to sleep and recovered.

NEURALGIA. — TIC DOLOUREUX.

An acute darting pain in the course of some of the nerves, occurring in paroxysms, produced by the slightest touch, and without general fever, characterises this disease.

Its history is interesting and instructive. Though it is now one of the most common diseases, yet the first published account we find of it, is that of M. Andre of Versailles in 1756. Seventeen years after this, (1773) Dr. Fothergill communicated to the London Medical Society, some remarks on this disease, to which he gave the name of "a painful affection of the face." Fothergill was not aware that any one had described it before himself; and in fact, the credit of making known the disease to the medical world, is due to him, as he it was, who first described it with such accuracy, as to enable others to recognise it, as a distinct disease.

Though this painful disease is now so common in this country, that there are few physicians who have not seen many cases of it, yet it seems it was scarcely known here, thirty years ago. How is this to be accounted for? Evidence of its being quite a recent disease in this country, is as follows. In 1806 Dr. Gardner Jones, a respectable physician in New York, was attacked by Tic Doloureux of the face. In 1809, he wrote an account of his sufferings to Dr. Rush, of Philadelphia, in which he says, "Of all the medical gentlemen with whom I have conversed respecting my complaint, only *one* has professed ever to have seen a case of the disease prior to my own; nor can I recollect more than two who could recognise its singular features as described in any author they had read. To most practitioners, even those of eminence, the name itself is a perfect novelty. Since the attention of our physicians has been directed to this subject, one other case, but of much less asperity and poignancy than my own has been detected here." Dr. Rush recommended the use of belladonna and stramonium, but it is a singular fact, that neither of these, now common remedies, could be procured in New York. "I was disposed," says Dr. Jones, "to have tried them, and for this purpose took great pains to procure them, but ineffectually, as these articles were not to be found with the druggists or apothecaries, being seldom used in the practice of our physicians."*

The disease has also greatly increased within a few years in other countries, "this distressing disease," says Dr. James Johnson, "becomes more common every day, and is on the increase, with a host of other nervous affections." Dr. Baillie observes, "that it has become more common of late years."

The *exciting causes* of Neuralgia, are various. Exposure to wet and cold is the most common. Malaria, as has been ably shown by Dr. Macculloch, frequently gives rise to it. Stretching, pressure, or other injuries of the nerves, carious teeth, disorder of the stomach, or alimentary canal, or of the uterus, and spinal irritation also cause this disease.

---

* The Philadelphia Medical Museum, Vol. 1, New Series, 1811.

Pathology. — It will not be disputed that the seat of this disease is in the nervous system, but at what point, it is difficult to determine. Not always in the nerve at the place of the pain, for the disease may exist for years, without any perceptible alteration in the nerve. Sir Henry Halford, thinks that its most awful form, affecting the branches of the fifth pair of nerves, is caused by diseased bone. He refers to a case arising from exostosis of the alveolar process, another from disease of the antrum highmorianum, and another from a tumour on the internal surface of the skull. Other cases might be referred to, in corroboration of this opinion.

A late writer, Dr. Osborne, in the *Dublin Journal* of *Medical Sciences*, Nov. 1837, attributes the disease, to a partial paralysis of a nerve, sufficient to alter its mode of sensation, but not to obliterate it.

Many cases of Neuralgia arise from some local injury of a nerve ; here the cause is obvious ; but in other cases the origin and the seat of the disease are quite obscure. I am induced to believe that in such cases, the seat of the disease is most generally in the brain. The worst cases I have ever known, or of which I have heard, those that after harrassing persons with indescribable suffering and terminating fatally, have been found connected with organic disease of the brain. A deplorable case of this kind which I witnessed arose from a tumour at the base of brain. Innumerable are the pains in various parts of the body, which patients, laboring under disease of the brain, complain of, before any affection of this organ is suspected. Such patients attribute all their sufferings to disease of the part where the pain is, or to the stomach, which is often affected by nausea. Andral mentions a case of ramollissment of the brain, going on for a considerable time, while the only symptom of disease, was pain in the lower extremities.

23*

I do not suppose that organic lesion will always be found in the brain, in cases of Neuralgia that originate there. The disease is no doubt merely functional in many cases, or the change in that portion of the cerebral structure destined to sensibility, and which change causes the disease, may not be obvious to our senses.

Many cases of Neuralgia seem to arise from a highly irritable and excitable state of the nervous system. Some of these, are attributed to slight injuries, to a sprain, or bruise, or puncture. They continue, at intervals, for a long time, reproduced and kept up, by mental emotion, perhaps by the mental attention directed to the injured part. I have known a young lady suffer severely from intermittent neuralgia, affecting one of her fingers. Any excitement of mind, or any unusual mental effort when she was free from pain, would immediately reproduce it.

But often the severest pain is in a part which has received no injury Such cases must arise from disease of the nervous system at some other point, either of the brain or in the course of the nerves that supply the painful part. Injury of a nerve in its course often produces pain, no where but at the extremity of the nerve. After amputations, patients complain of pain in the fingers and toes of the amputated limbs.

The following is one of the most interesting and instructive cases of this kind, of which I have ever heard : — *It is from Hennen.*

CASE LXI. — " A general officer, of distinguished gallantry, was struck by a round shot during a very desperately fought action, which buffing along his breast in an oblique direction, destroyed the arm, and left only the head of the bone and a very small portion of the shaft remaining. He was carried to an adjoining hovel, where the common amputation was performed under very unfavorable circumstances; the night was coming on, the supply of candles was scanty, and the enemy's shot were flying in all directions. The general was placed under my care on the day after the operation. The variety of cross accidents from fever and extensive sloughing, it is not within my purpose at present to enlarge upon, but the first attempt at clearing the ligatures, and making gentle pressure on them, was attended with pain so excruciating, as to leave no doubt that each included a nerve, or was in a certain degree connected with some large nervous filaments. This agonizing sensation was not felt except the ligatures were pulled at, and then not in the stump itself, but was referred to the finger, thumb, wrist, elbow, or even to the external skin of the lost arm, as one or other ligature might be handled. I have sometimes been led to think, that the general uniformly felt the same sensations when the same ligature was touched, as I generally made my attempts to extricate them in a regulated succession, and his complaints were often in the same succession of parts. More attentive observation, however, convinced me that this was not the case; for if any one was pulled with more steadiness than the other, he complained of all the parts, suffering pain simultaneously. One small ligature, if pulled in an oblique direction *inwards* towards the axilla, always gave him imaginary pain about the elbow or in the skin; but if the same was pulled strongly and directly *downwards*, the fingers were complained of. He has, frequently, after the smarting of dressing was over, with great accuracy pointed out on my arm the course of the internal cutaneous nerve, as the site of his ideal pain; often he has described that of the external : and, on one occasion, I, with utter astonishment, had the general neurology of my arm and fingers traced by him. But unless the ligatures were pulled at, he had no other uneasy sensations than those which usually occur in persons whose limbs have been amputated. Once only did I ever know him refer his pain to the seat of the sensorium itself. On that occasion, from using an artery forceps to the ligatures, on which the slide moved rather stiffly, I exerted a greater force than I had intended. He convulsively put his hand to his head, expressed a sense of exquisite pain in his brain, involuntary tears dropped from his eyes, a paralytic contraction momentarily affected his mouth, a universal paleness spread over the uncovered parts of his body ; and, although unusually tolerant of pain, and of a most remarkable equanimity of temper, he uttered a piercing cry, and exclaimed, " that the agony in his head and neck was insufferable." The state of the collapse was so great, that I was obliged to send an aid-de-camp instantly for volatile alkali, and a glass of Maderia, by which he was soon relieved ; but the painful sensation, and the prostration of his strength, continued through the day. A British admiral was present on this and various other occasions, and observed to me, after I had confessed my inability to explain, even to my own satisfaction, the cause of all these sensations, " that he never saw the general dressed without applying mentally to the wonderful sympathy manifested on those occasions, the expression of Pope : 'it lives along the line.'" I believe we must be content with the fact, without seeking for the explanation."

Treatment. — Some cases, have, for a while, at least, been relieved by surgical operations ; by cutting off the nervous communication between the painful part and the brain. See Case XLVI, p. 166.

I have had recourse to this method in a few cases, but without permanent benefit, and on a review of the accounts published of this plan of treatment, we do not find it often successful. Still cases occur, no doubt, in which recourse to it would be proper.

Applications to the painful part quite frequently afford relief. A hot solution of Sugar of Lead and Laudanum, and very hot water applied for a considerable time to the painful nerves, I have known remove the pain entirely. A plaster of equal parts of Extract of Belladonna and Soap Cerate, sometimes has the same effect.

I have seen Veratria and Aconitine used in cases of great severity. An ointment made of 20 grains of Veratria to an ounce of lard, for awhile, gave almost complete relief. About half a drachm was rubbed over the painful part three or four times a day. Its effects were immediate and soothing. After a few days, however, it ceased to have any good effect and was discontinued. It is used for a like purpose dissolved in hot alcohol. Ten to thirty grains of Veratria to an ounce of alcohol. This is rubbed on the skin, and produces no soreness unless the skin is very irritable. It causes, however, a tingling heat, which for a while relieves the neuralgic pain. Veratria is also given internally. Turnbull uses the following pill.

R. Veratriæ, . . . gr. ii.
Pulv. Rad. Glycyrrh, . gr. xii.
Ext. Hyoscyam, . . gr. vi.

Make into twelve pills, one of which may be taken three times a day. If there is a tendency to Costiveness, a few grains of compound rhubarb pill, may be substituted for the two last ingredients.

Aconitine has also been used for this disease. A late number of the Lancet, Jan. 6th, 1838, contains a notice by the Rev. Sidney Smith, of a severe case of *tic douloureux*, of seven years' standing, which was cured for eight weeks, to the date of the report, by the use of the Aconitine ointment — one grain to a drachm of lard.

I have used Granville's Counter-Irritant, or the strongest Liquor Ammoniæ, in several cases; but in none has it afforded relief for more than half an hour. The pain in one case was aggravated by it.

Constitutional remedies have with me been more useful. I have derived the most benefit from Carbonate of Iron in large doses; from one to four drachms, four times a day, usually combined with pulverised cinnamon or ginger, and care being taken not to have it accumulate in the bowels. Arsenic is often very serviceable. I consider it one of the best of remedies in this disease. I have used Fowler's Solution, but prefer the following pill, the formula of which will be found in the second volume of the Asiatic Researches. Take of recent white arsenic *thirteen* grains, black pepper, *seventy-eight* grains, beat in an iron mortar for four days at intervals, then remove to a stone mortar, and with water make *one hundred* pills. Dose *one*, two or three times a day.

Peruvian Bark and Quinine are efficacious remedies in intermittent neuralgia.

The Extract of Conium, in large doses, has sometimes afforded relief and effected a cure when other remedies have failed. A medical friend had this disease in its most agonizing form, chiefly affecting the lower jaw. He took large doses of opium without any mitigation of his suffering, and without producing a tendency to sleep. He then had recourse to Extract of Conium, of which he took half an ounce in the course of a night. This afforded relief and seemingly affected a cure, as he has not been troubled with it for several years.

Dr. James Jackson, of Boston, cured a severe case of this disease by the same remedy. He gave in the course of six hours, sixty pills of Extract of Conium, making three hundred grains.*

---

* The New England Journal of Medicine and Surgery, Vol. 2.

M. Jolly, in the article, *Nevralgie, Dictionnaire de Medicine et de Chirurgie Pratiques*, recommends the following:

> R. Ferri. Carb. Praep., . oz. ss.
> Sulph. Quinine, . . grs. xvi.
> Opium, . . . grs. iv.

Mix and divide into sixteen powders, one of which is to be given every six hours.

> R. Ferrocyanate of Iron, . grs. xviii.
> Sulph. Quinine, . . grs. xii.
> Opium, ... grs. ii.

Make into twelve pills with conserve of roses, and give one three times a day.

He also recommends the following sternutory, in Neuralgia of the face. Red Bark, (*Cinchona rubra,*) and common snuff, equal parts.

I have used with good effect in similar cases a snuff made of one drachm of common snuff, four grains of Quinine, and a quarter of a grain of Morphine.

It has already been mentioned, page 148, that **Mr.** Teale supposes many cases of Neuralgia arise from irritation of the Spinal marrow. In such cases he states there is tenderness over some of the Vertebrae, and leeching and blistering afford relief.

An eruption on the skin, like nettle rash, has been known to remove the pain immediately.

DYSPEPSIA.

In a previous work, "Remarks on the influence of Mental Cultivation and Mental Excitement upon health," I stated my opinion that "a majority of the cases of Dyspepsia, especially among students, arose from disease of the brain and nervous system, and were perpetuated by mental excitement."

Subsequent observation has confirmed me in the correctness of this opinion. Dyspepsia is a disease peculiar to man and to civilized man. Why is this so? Some say because he pampers his appetite by numerous dishes and eats too much. But other animals than man, and men in an uncivilized state, savages and barbarians, eat, especially at times, much more than men in civilized countries, yet they digest what they eat without difficulty. Besides it is not true, that dyspepsia is confined to those who live luxuriously, who daily eat the richest and most nutritious food and drink good wine. The worst cases occur in students, clergymen, and those who have for the most part lived on plain food.

The reason why civilized man is most subject to indigestion, is to me obvious. Every one knows that excitement and anxiety of mind impairs the appetite, and hinders digestion. This mental agitation consumes, or hinders the transmission of the nervous fluid or nervous power from the brain to the stomach, that is necessary to create an appetite, and to complete digestion. The same cause prevents the proper secretion of bile, and renders the bowels torpid.

It is true that a full meal sometimes produces a severe attack of dyspepsia in one thus disposed to it. It is however, because the stomach, from the cause above stated, is not able to digest it.

Hence, those thus inclined to dyspepsia, must pursue one of two courses in order to prevent its attacks.

They must either free themselves from anxiety and care, and avoid fatiguing mental labor, or else they must live quite sparingly and on unstimulating food. If they consume the nervous fluid or energy, in labor of the brain, they must require but little labor of the stomach. Not only the stomach, but every part of the body becomes disordered, when thus robbed by the brain of their due proportion of nervous power. Thus we find in such individuals, there is not enough of this nervous power to heal wounds and other injuries of the body readily.

Injury of nerves, that derange or cut off the communication between the brain and the parts supplied by the injured nerves, produces atrophy of these parts. Thus Lobstein, relates the case of a man, aged 54, whose right leg ceased to grow, after an injury of the crural and sciatic nerves, received when a child.

When the stomach becomes deranged from the cause mentioned, other organs as the liver, lungs, uterus, skin, &c., also become disordered from what is called sympathy. This sympathy is not, however, direct between the organs, but takes place through the brain; for all the sympathies depend on changes in this organ. In this way, and only in this way, do the viscera sympathise, and not by means of direct nervous connexion. When the brain has been overtasked and over-excited, then these sympathetic disorders are seen to increase.

Now and then we are told of an individual, whose mental labors are great and who enjoys good health. In such instances the mental labor though it would be great and fatiguing to many, is not so to the individual. His large and well proportioned brain, accomplishes with ease, what would be exhausting labor to another, just as a man of largely developed muscular powers, will accomplish without fatigue what would prove severely injurious to one whose muscular system was small and delicate.

But we daily see numerous instances of men, who have never been dyspeptic, and we also see many who

24

are almost constantly so. The first class is composed
for the most part, of men of happy temperaments, men
who have but little anxiety of mind, who are seldom
long perplexed by any occurrence. These men have a
good appetite, and indulge it ; they eat each meal with
enjoyment, and slowly, and without a thought, or any
apprehension of distress from it.

The other class is made up of a very different kind of
men — men who are never so free from care — the per-
plexities of business, or some kind of mental anxiety, as
to be able to eat their meals slowly and happily. Among
this class are to be found many who are so fearful of
sinning against some theory of which they have heard
or read, about the danger of eating animal food, puddings,
pies, &c. ; or of drinking coffee, tea, or a glass of wine ; or
of omitting to eat bran bread and to drink cold water, that
their minds are perpetually agitated before and during
their meals, and afterwards occupied in watching and
waiting for some sensations from the stomach to enable
them to determine whether the meal is injurious or not.

This class of persons are sure to complain of disorder
of the stomach, if they indulge in any other than the most
mild food, and in small quantity. Feeling disordered
after a full meal or after having eaten of some rich food,
they attribute their bad feelings to the food they have
just taken, when in fact, it ought to be attributed to the
brain having robbed the stomach of that nervous power
essential to carry on digestion.

I do not mean to say that Dyspepsia always originates
in this way. Undoubtedly, it frequently arises from primary disease of the stomach. But I mean to say that
numerous cases of this disease arise from primary disorder of the brain, which disorder is the result of mental
agitation. Is it not owing to this cause that the disease

prevails among mankind and not among other animals, and that it is more common in enlightened than in unenlightened communities ?

As the disease, of itself, is seldom fatal, we do not often have an opportunity of calling to our aid post mortem researches, in determining its seat. There are some cases, however, of death from what was considered dyspepsia, where examination after death tended to confirm the view we have taken of this disease. I have already stated that disease of the cerebellum very frequently gave rise to dyspeptic symptoms. Case XIII, page 78, and Case XVII, page 86, and Case XXI, page 96, are instances of this.

Two of the worst cases I have known, of Dyspepsia, and which were considered and treated by several physicians as such for a period of seven or eight years, exhibited at length unequivocal symptoms of disorder of the brain. One has become deranged, the other has now epileptic fits. It may be said that disorder of the stomach produced the disease of the brain. I think this was not the case, for both the individuals had undergone much mental anxiety previous to their dyspeptic symptoms, and were themselves of the opinion that this caused the disorder of the stomach.

Some years since, a young gentleman, became from some unknown cause, quite dyspeptic. His stomach was very irritable, and for a considerable time even a small quantity of mild food would occasion distress and flatulence of the stomach, or it would be rejected.

A cough, and symptoms of disease of the lungs ensued, and it was considered a case of latent or dyspeptic phthisis. Soon after, mental derangement occurred, and the patient remained insane for two years when he died. I was not present at the post mortem examination, but have been assured by a physician who was, that there was no disease of the stomach, and but little of the lungs, but that the brain was greatly disorganised.

I might quote from the works of medical writers numerous cases where dissection of those long considered dyspeptic, who complained only of the stomach, exhibited no disease of this organ, while the brain was found considerably diseased. Several such cases will be found in a late work by Dr. Wilson Philip.* He mentions the case of a student at Oxford, whose complaint was regarded by his physicians, of that place, and of London, as dyspepsia, but which finally proved fatal, and on examination after death, but trifling marks of disease were found, except at the base of the brain, and in the cerebellum and medulla oblongata. Dr. Darwall, in an interesting paper on "Some forms of cerebral and spinal irritation," furnished several cases in support of his views that indigestion does not merely influence the nervous system, but that the nervous system is the source from which the indigestion proceeds.

"Dr. Abercrombie, on *Organic Diseases of the Brian*, says, that 'Symptoms which really depend upon disease of the brain, are very apt to be referred to the stomach.' After mentioning several cases, in which for a long time the prominent symptoms were those of dyspepsia, and in which no trace of organic disease of the stomach was discovered after death, but tumors, or other disease of the brain, he says, 'Many other cases of organic disease of the brain are on record, in which the only morbid appearances were in the head, though some of the most prominent symptoms had been in the stomach. Some of these resembled what has been called sick-headache,

---

* A Treatise on the more obscure Affections of the Brain, &c., by A. P. W. Philip, M. D.

others were chiefly distinguished by remarkable distur-
bances of the digestive functions.' Dr. A. adds this important caution; — 'In cases of this class we must
beware of being misled, in regard to the nature of the
complaint, by observing that the symptoms in the stomach are alleviated by attention to regimen, or by treatment directed to the stomach itself. If digestion be
impeded, from whatever cause, these uneasy symptoms
in the stomach may be alleviated by great attention to
diet, but no inference can be drawn from this source, in
regard to the cause of the derangement.'

This last quotation, I think explains a very common
mistake — a mistake which is not only made by dyspeptics themselves, but by writers on this disease. They
suppose because *low diet*, &c. relieves the principal
symptoms in the stomach, that therefore the disease is
confined to that organ; when in fact the disease is in
the head, but is manifested only by the stomach, the liver,
or some organ with which the brain sympathises, and the
low diet gives relief, by lessening the too energetic action
of the brain.

Dr. Hastings, of England, has called attention to this
subject, in the *Midland Medical and Surgical Register*
of 1831. He says, that not unfrequently cases occur,
which exhibit symptoms of disordered stomach, accompanied by increased determination of blood to the head,
alternate flushings and coldness, irregular spirits, &c.;
and he states that in all the cases which terminated
fatally, under his care, he found thickening of the membranes of the brain, and marks of chronic inflammation
within the head. Dr. H. believes that many of the nervous symptoms of which dyspeptic persons complain,
are produced by slow alteration of the brain, in consequence of chronic inflammation; and recommends

24*

leeches, cold applications to the head, and issues in the neck, for the relief of such cases.

M. Bayle has published in the *Revue Medicale*, several cases, exhibiting the connexion between disease of the brain and disorder of the stomach. He endeavors to show that disease of the stomach often produces insanity; but he mentions that many of his patients were remarkable for violent temper, or were melancholy, or exhibited some symptoms of nervous irritation, before they were much unwell; then the stomach became disordered, and finally derangement of the mind ensued. On dissection, the brain and its membranes were found diseased; and here I apprehend was the original seat of the complaint, (produced probably by some moral cause,) which first manifested itself in change of temper, or slight nervous affections; then, as it increased, disordered the stomach by sympathy, and finally produced so much disease of the brain as to cause insanity.

Dr. Burrows relates the case of a lady, who had been unwell for several years. She referred all her suffering to the stomach. and often said, that when she was dead, *there* would be found the seat of the disease. She died rather suddenly with fever and delirium, after exposure in a very hot day; and on examining the body, no trace of disease appeared in the stomach or bowels, but the brain exhibited marks of *long standing disease.**

Some cases and observations in a late work of M. Barras,† confirm the opinion I have advanced respecting the cause and seat of dyspepsia, though this writer does not believe, with M. Broussais and others, that it is an

---

* Burrows on Insanity, p. 236.

† Traite sur les Gastralgies et les Enteralgies, ou Maladies Nerveu-se de l'Estomac et des Intestins. Par J. P. T. Barras, M. D.

inflammatory disease, but that it consists in an affection of the nerves of the stomach, or what Dr. Johnson calls *morbid sensibility* of the stomach, bowels, &c. He considers the disease to be a *gastralgia*, and not gastritis. But what causes this gastralgia, or morbid sensibility of the stomach? An attentive examination of the cases he has cited, will show that, very probably, the first cause of morbid action was a *moral one.* Most of the patients whose cases he relates, were of an irritable, nervous temperament, and previous to any symptoms of disease of the stomach, they had 'experienced severe domestic affliction,' had been 'melancholy,' or been afflicted by 'great mental suffering,' or had 'studied severely, or been exposed to constant turmoils.'

One case terminated fatally. It was that of a lady 56 years of age, who had been subject to mental sufferings, and constantly complained of pain in the region of the stomach. Her physician predicted that disorder of the stomach would be found, but on examination no disease of this organ was seen, but there was serous effusion into the ventricles of the brain.

The following is a case which terminated favorably, and which M. Barras regards as primarily a disorder of the stomach. I believe it to have been from the first a functional disease of the brain. It is very similar to many cases that terminate in insanity, and I have no doubt this would, if the depleting plan of treatment had been continued, instead of that proposed by M. Barras.

CASE LXII.—"Madam C., aged 43 years, of very nervous temperament, and subject to pains in her stomach, experienced a severe domestic affliction, in September, 1825. Immediately afterwards, the gastric affection was much aggravated, accompanied by spasms in the chest and sense of suffocation. For these, leeches were thrice applied, mucilaginous drinks prescribed, and the most rigorous regimen enjoined. In November, she became affected with furious delirium, and in this state, she craved lustily for animal food, and sought to obtain it by main force. M. Barras was consulted, and advised that better nourishment should be allowed. The digestion was distressing at first; but, by gradually habituating the stomach to animal matters, the digestion became easy, and, by the 15th December, the patient could drink a bottle of Bordeaux wine without inconvenience. With this power of receiving aliment, the strength and flesh returned—her mental aberration disappeared in a great measure, and there is every appearance of complete recovery."

Treatment.— In every case of Dyspepsia, it is important to investigate the condition of the brain; at the same time, that of the stomach, liver and other organs should not be overlooked. In some cases attention to those last organs is all that is required. Mercurial remedies are usually injurious, but in some rare instances when the liver is disordered, a few doses of blue pill may be of much service. Combinations of laxatives and tonics with alkalies are frequently useful. The preparations of iron, quinine or some of the vegetable bitters, combined with rhubarb or aloes, in such proportions as to give tone to the stomach and bowels, and to insure their regular action, are often very beneficial. But a very large class of dyspeptics, especially those who have long suffered from disorders of the stomach, should be advised to seek restoration to health, not in the daily use of medicines, or in an unusual course of diet, but in judicious exertion of the body. in travelling through countries where the mind will be pleasantly occupied, in innocent amusements, cheerful company, ordinary diet, inattention to their stomachs, and *mental relaxation.*

Where there is reason to apprehend organic disease of the brain, moxas, setons in the neck and cupping should be resorted to.

INSANITY.

The article on Insanity in the North American Review, for January, 1837, and in the American Journal of the Medical Sciences for November, 1838, the former being a review of Prichard, and the latter of Esquirol on Insanity, were prepared by the author of this work. To those articles he refers the reader, for details respecting this interesting disease that will not be found in this chapter.

The following table, made up from the statements of Esquirol, M. Briere de Boismont and other good authorities exhibits, perhaps, as accurate an account of the number of the insane in different countries, and in the large cities of Europe, as can at present be obtained.

COUNTRIES.	POPULATION.	NO. OF INSANE.	PROPORTION.
England,	12,700,000	16.222	793
Scotland,	2,093,500	3.652	563
France,	32,000,000	32,000	1.000
Norway,	1,051,300	1,909	551
Belgium,	3,816,000	3,763	1,014
Holland,	2,302,000	2,300	1,046
Italy,	16,789,000	1,441	4,879
Spain,	4,085,000	569	7,181
U. States,*	12,866,020	16,000	800
Westphalia,			846
Saxony,			968

* The above estimate of the number of the insane is to a considerable degree, conjectural. In the next census for this country, lunatics and idiots are to be included.

CITIES.	POPULATION.	NO. OF INSANE.	PROPORTION.
London,	1,400,000	7,000	200
Paris,	890,000	4,000	222
Petersburg,	377,000	120	3,133
Naples,	370,000	479	759
Cairo,	330,000	14	30,714
Madrid,	204,000	60	3,350
Rome,	154,000	320	481
Milan,	151,000	618	242
Turin,	114,000	331	344
Florence,	80,000	236	338
Dresden.	70,000	150	466

From the above table we learn that this disease, more frequently occurs in large cities than in the country : and that it prevails the most in enlightened and educated communities In fact, insanity is almost wholly confined to the civilized races of men. It is rare among the uncivilized and uneducated Indians and Negroes. It is uncommon in China, Persia, Hindostan, Turkey and Russia. There is but little in Spain and Portugal, while it prevails to a great extent in England, France, Germany, Norway, Holland, and in the United States. In these last countries, it is thought by those who have investigated the subject, to have considerably increased, within the last half century. This fact, says M. Belhomme, cannot be doubted.

Causes of Insanity. — A very common division of the causes of insanity, is into moral and physical. Modern writers, do not. however, agree as to the comparative influence of these causes. This arises from some having included among physical causes, hereditary predisposition and certain diseases, which others do not consider as properly belonging to this class.

Most writers, however, attach the greatest importance to moral causes. " The observations," says M. Georget, " which I have had in my power to make, the more numerous ones which I have compared in authors, have convinced me, that, among one hundred lunatics, ninety-five at least have become such from the influence of affections and of moral commotions : it is an obser-. vation become almost proverbial in the hospital — the Salpetriere, — 'qu'on perd la tete par les revolutions d'esprit.' The first question that M. Pinel puts to a new patient who still preserves some remains of intelligence, is, Have you undergone any vexation or disappointment? Seldom is the reply in the negative. " It is," continues the same writer, " in the age in which the mind is most susceptible of strong feelings, in which the passions are excited by the strongest interests, that madness is principally displayed. Children, calm and without anxiety, incapable of long and extensive combinations of thought, not yet initiated into the troubles of life, and old men, whom the now vanishing illusions of their preceding age, and their increasing physical and moral weakness render indifferent as to events, are but rarely affected. The same remark applies to persons who in their constitution approach to the character of children or of old men."*

It may also be urged in favor of this opinion, that the disease is comparatively rare among uncultivated nations; though they are exposed to the same physical causes.

I fully concur in the opinion of M. Georget, that moral causes are far more operative in the production of this disease, than physical ones ; and it appears to me, that those who have come to a different conclusion, have placed under the head of physical causes, many that ought not to be thus included.

---

* De la Folie, par M. Georget, &c., Paris, 1820.

Hereditary predisposition, cerebral diseases, as apoplexy, palsy and epilepsy; ill health, dyspepsia, bodily disorder and masturbation, are by some considered physical causes of insanity. But it appears to me, they do not properly belong to this class.

Hereditary predisposition to insanity, consists, for the most part, in a peculiarity in the structure of the brain, which is transmitted from parents. But it is not a peculiarity, or defective formation of the brain, wholly confined to those whose parents or ancestors were insane; neither is it disease, nor would it lead to insanity, without the agency of moral causes.

As for Apoplexy, Palsy, Epilepsy, Dyspepsia, &c., they are produced by moral causes, and are the first symptoms of disordered brain manifested by some, who become insane. Most insane persons have dyspepsia, or some bodily disorder, previous to becoming mentally deranged. They have slight disease of the brain, produced I apprehend, generally, by circumstances affecting and agitating the mind. This slight disease of the brain is sufficient to impair the functions of the stomach or the functions of other organs. After a while the disease of the brain increases so as to derange the mental faculties, and then not unfrequently the dyspepsia or other bodily disorder disappears. This is, I believe, in most cases, the true explanation of the bodily disorder that precedes insanity.

Masturbation is assigned as a physical cause of insanity. I presume that some cases originate from the practice of this vice, though I consider it, rather a moral than a physical cause. Uncontrollable mental emotion induces a resort to it. But I much doubt its being a frequent cause. I am aware that the insane are frequently seen to practise it, and I know that in them, it has sometimes at least, most baneful effects; hurrying them on to idiocy and death; but generally I regard it as the effect of the disease of the brain, which causes the insanity.

I have often conversed with a gentleman, who has several times been an inmate of a Lunatic Hospital for periodical insanity. He has assured me that each attack was preceded by an uncontrollable desire to gratify himself by the indulgence of this propensity, and this desire continued during his insanity, but ceased with it. So strong was it, he said, that nothing, — even the knowledge that instant death was to follow, would have been sufficient to have deterred him from resorting to it. A few years since I caused much inquiry upon this subject to be made at the Connecticut State Prison. I ascertained that there was scarcely an instance of a prisoner who did not practice it. Many of them had for years, and some of them daily. I have no doubt it is a very common practice among prisoners, yet we seldom hear of one becoming insane from this cause. I never have heard of a single instance.

The moral causes of this disease are very numerous. They vary in different countries and at different eras. They are such as, Pecuniary embarrasments, Domestic griefs, Over exertion of mind, Religious anxiety, Political events, Disappointment in love, Disappointed ambition, Erroneous education, &c.

In all countries there is an increase of insanity, from moral causes, — by events that excite deep and general feeling among the inhabitants. Dr. Macdonald, late resident Physician of the Bloomingdale Asylum, in an interesting article on the statistics of that Institution, in the October number of the *New-York Journal of Medicine and Surgery*, says, " within the writer's own experience, the Anti-Masonic excitement, the Jackson excitement, and the Anti-Jackson excitement, the Bank excitement,

25

the Abolition excitement, and the Speculating excitement, have each furnished the Asylum with inmates."

The French Revolution increased it in France, the American Revolution in this country. The reformation of Luther, the noted South Sea Speculation in England about 1720, and the wars of Bonaparte, augmented the number of insane. When Napoleon made and unmade kings and queens with great rapidity, kings and queens increased in the mad houses of France. When the Pope came to Paris, an event that excited the religious community of that country, cases of religious insanity became more numerous. "So great has been the influence of our political commotions," says Esquirol, "that I could give the history of France from the taking of the Bastile to the last appearance of Bonaparte, by that of the insane of the hospitals, whose delusions related to the different events of that long period of history."

Erroneous modes of education are, we apprehend, very powerful in increasing the susceptibility to mental derangement. "There are two different points of view," says Prichard, in his excellent Treatise on Insanity, "under which the injurious effects of wrong education may be considered. By too great indulgence and a want of moral discipline, the passions acquire great power, and a character is formed subject to caprice and to violent emotions : a predisposition to Insanity is thus laid in the temper and moral affections of the individual. An over-strained and premature exercise of the intellectual powers, is likewise a fault of education which predisposes to insanity as it does to all other diseases of the brain."

Other causes which appear to be quite operative in producing insanity, especially of late years, and in this country, deserve notice.

Intoxicating liquors. — The immoderate use of in-

toxicating drinks is a much more frequent cause of insanity in the United States, in England, Ireland, and
Germany, than in France, Italy, and in Spain.   Of 1264
lunatics admitted into the Charenton, Paris, from 1826
to 1833, 134 were rendered insane from the use of intoxicating drinks; a far greater number in proportion
than were attributed to this cause in previous years.
Esquirol says, that in his private establishment for the
insane, out of 330 lunatics, in only *three* could the disease
be attributed to the use of stimulating drinks, and one of
these he believed became intemperate in consequence of
insanity.

" In the public Lunatic Asylums in England," says Dr.
Prichard, "it is generally known that, in a great proportion of cases, dram-drinking is the exciting cause of the
insanity."   In the Richmond Lunatic Asylum, Dublin,
one-fifth of all the cases are caused by intoxication.   Of
608 insane persons at this institution, 74 men and 12
women were supposed to have become mentally deranged from this cause.

In the Massachusetts State Lunatic Hospital, at Wor-
cester, according to the late able and interesting report
of the superintendant, Dr. Woodward, about one-fifth of
the cases are attributed to this cause, or 158 out of 855.
Of the 152 cases of periodical insanity that have been in
the hospital 94 or nearly two thirds of the whole have
arrisen from intemperance.   But it should be recollected
that this excellent hospital is for pauper lunatics; other
asylums for the insane in this country do not receive so
large a proportion of patients rendered insane by intemperance.   At the Connecticut Retreat for the Insane, at
Hartford, of 116 patients only *two* are stated in the report for 1834, to have been rendered insane by "intemperance," and *two* others by "dissipation and exhausta-
tion, consequent upon dissipation."

Pathology. — I have in other parts of this work, particularly at page 57, referred to the latest researches respecting the condition of the brain in insanity.   The
writings of Foville, Calmeil, Falret and Bayle, are high
authority on this subject.   The results of their researches may be principally summed up as follows.

1st. In mental alienation the brain invariably presents lesions which can be distinctly recognized.   Exceptions to this, if ever observed, are extremely rare.

2nd. These lesions vary according to the acute or
chronic form of the malady, and according to the character of the affection, whether simple, confined to intellectual disorder merely, or complicated with disorder
of sensation and motion.

3d. In simple intellectual derangement of an acute
or recent character, the grey cortical substance of the
cerebral convolutions is altered in color and consistence.
It is red, marbled ecchymosed and indurated.   In chronic cases all these appearances are more marked.   The
external cortical layer in such may be seperated like a
membrane from the lower stratum.   In the very chronic cases, especially in dementia, there is often atrophy of
the grey substance of the cerebral convolutions.

4th. In intellectual derangement complicated with derangement of motion, with paralysis more or less general ; in addition to the alterations of the grey substance
already noticed, there are lesions of the white substance
or medullary portion of the brain.   These are, either
hardening, serous infiltration or softening and generally
morbid adhesions of the fibres of the medullary portion
of the brain.

These views respecting the pathology of insanity, are
borne out by numerous facts and cases ; a considerable
number of which, have already been related in this work.

They are also in accordance with the recent brilliant researches in embryology and comparative anatomy — researches that lead us to regard the grey substance of the brain as the seat of the intellect. In fœtal life this portion of the brain is deficient, — it appears with the first manifestations of intellect. Among animals we notice its increase, as we ascend in the scale of animal organization.

It is to be hoped, and I think expected, that further researches, respecting the diseases of the brain, will enable us to know, in many cases, from the symptoms, what part of this organ is affected. Some cases have already been adduced, rendering this not improbable. A considerable number of facts and cases bearing upon this subject have been collected by phrenological writers. These should not be disregarded, and in every case of disease of the brain the phrenological system should be kept in view. If this system is correct, and pathological researches can determine if it is so, it must surely be of great service in the treatment of the diseases of the brain.

Prevention. - Methods of prevention are obvious ; consisting for the most part, in carefully guarding against unduly tasking and exciting the minds of children ; in avoiding through life, as much as possible, every thing likely to produce long continued and severe mental harassment ; and in preventing those predisposed to the disease, from marrying and transmitting it, to their offspring. It is the imperative duty of physicians, and of every well wisher to the human race, to use all their influence, to prevent intermarriages in familes where insanity is known to be hereditary.

Treatment. — This is, with propriety, divided into the
25*

Medical or Therapeutical, and the Moral. We shall
very briefly treat of both.

First, of the Medical or Therapeutical treatment of
the Insane.

The greatest error I have seen committed in the
medical treatment of the insane, is the neglect of depletion in the early stage, and of narcotics and tonics in
the subsequent. At the commencement of a considerable portion of the cases of insanity, there is an inflammatory condition of the brain or of its membranes, or
if not actual inflammation, there is very considerable
vascular excitement of these structures, and depletion
will sometimes arrest the disease, the same as it will
pneumonia. Bleeding, and antimonials and the antiphlogistic treatment generally, are then serviceable.

But soon this state terminates in death or in a morbid
condition of the brain, in an irritable state of this organ,
probably somewhat resembling that in delirium tremens.
Then opiates and other narcotics are serviceable. In
most cases it is well to commence the use of them with
caution, giving but small doses at first. Even, when
narcotics, in such cases, do not tend to cure, they often
produce some abatement in the violence of the maniacal
paroxysms and ensure a beneficial degree of calmness
that could not be obtained without them. Many cases
of mania, especially of intermittent mania, are much
benefitted by tonics, by quinine, arsenic, and the preparations of iron.

Some practitioners having cured a few cases by bleeding, purgatives, &c., conclude that this is the proper
treatment for all ; while others, having seen injurious
effects result from depletion, and seen recoveries from
the use of narcotics and tonics, have concluded that
bleeding is improper in all cases, and tonics and narcotics
required in all.

I believe the cases that require depletion, especially by bleeding, are quite rare in comparison with those in which an opposite method of treatment is necessary. The advice of a physician is seldom sought, until there has been disease of the brain for a considerable time. A careful examination of most cases of insanity will show, that some disorder of the brain, existed for a time, often for a long time before the mental derangement was such as to attract particular attention. When disorder of the mind becomes obvious, the time has already passed in many cases for arresting the disease by bleeding, &c. The cases presented at Lunatic Hospitals seldom require reducing. Many of them have previous to their admission been injured by too copious abstractions of blood. Instead of requiring bleeding, they require nutritious food, tonics and narcotics.

In my opinion there is quite generally among practitioners of medicine, too great fear of opiates and narcotics, not only in insanity, but in all diseases of the head. One of the best chapters in the late work of Dr. Holland, " *Medical notes and reflection*," is, " on the use of opiates," in which this distinguished and experienced practioner, after remarking that opiates are now more largely employed than formerly, observes, that, " even now it may be affirmed that there exists a distrust, both as to the frequency and extent of their use, not warranted by facts, and injurious in various ways to our success in the treatment of disease."

He adds, in relation to the use of opium in cerebral affections, " there is great scope for further research on all that relates to disorders of the brain ; and a strong presumption that opium is capable here of larger and more beneficial application than has yet been given to it. In certain cases of insanity, especially where much active irritation is present without inflammation, its employment, not by partial and irregular doses, but by keeping the patient for some time steadily under its influence, is often attended with a good attainable in no other way. Here, as in so many cases of physical pain and irritation from other causes, the maintainance of repose is a summary advantage, giving time and power to the functions of the mind to resume their natural state."*

In some cases, full doses of opium will prove injurious, or be rejected from the stomach, while the same cases will be much benefited by this medicine when it is given in very small doses at first, and gradually increased. There are but few who will not bear this medicine when the use of it is thus conducted.

The great success that attended the treatment of the Insane, by my friend, the late Dr. Todd, at the *Connecticut Retreat for the Insane,* — a success unparalleled, must be ascribed, so far as the medical treatment had influence to the use of narcotics and tonics. In addition to the use of opium, he frequently employed other narcotics, as Conium, Hyoscyamus, Stramonium, &c. The extract of Conium with Iron was more frequently and more largely used by him than any other remedy. The following was a favorite prescription of his.

> R. Ferri Oxydum rub., . drachm, x.
> Ext. Conium, ... drachm, v.
> Syrup Bal. Tolu., . . oz. vi.
> Ol. Cinnam,
> Ol. Limon *a a*, . . . M. xii.
> Alcohol, ... oz. ii.
> Water, ... O. i.
> Brandy or Madeira Wine, O. ss.
> Sugar, ... oz. iv.—Mix.

---

* Dr. Seymour has well distinguished these cases, and made other valuable remarks in recommendation of opium. See cases of mental derangement, successfully treated by Acetate of Morphia. Medico-Chirurgical transactions, Vol. xix.

Of this he gave half an ounce, three or four times in a day.

Purgatives are sometimes very useful and in all cases a costive state of the bowels should be avoided. Both the warm and cold bath are occasionally serviceable. A great variety of other remedies have been recommonded, such as emetics, setons, moxas, the actual cautery, electricity, rotary machines, &c., &c. None of these are of much use generally, though there may be cases in which all, except the last, will be serviceable. Rotary machines are now considered useless in all cases, and dangerous in many.

Exercise of the body is one of the most essential remedial measures. Riding on horse-back, travelling to great distances amid new and interesting scenes, swimming, playing nine-pins, fencing, and gymnastic exercises, are all serviceable. The cultivation of the earth for some is the very best employment. Pinel advised that a farm should be attached to each lunatic hospital, to be cultivated by the patients. Bourgoin says that the poor insane at the hospital of Saragossa, Spain, cultivate the earth and are cured; while the rich, who will not labor, continue insane. Esquirol observes that the wealthy of either sex are not as much benefited by labor as the poor. He has, however, derived the best effects from the manual labor of the females at the Salpetriere; where they assemble in large rooms, and sew, knit, weave, &c.; while others have been benefited by attending to household duties, and others by cultivating a garden.

But there is no specific treatment of insanity. As its causes are various and combined, there must be a variety and combination of remedial measures.

Moral Treatment. — This, in many cases is more essential than the medical. Without judicious moral treatment, medical alone, will seldom affect a cure.

The first question that presents itself relates to the isolation of the insane, their *separation* from friends and home. Of the necessity of this, the physicians of all countries are agreed. The cases are rare that do not require separation from those with whom they live habitually. Willis observed that foreigners were more certainly cured in England than the natives; and Esquirol says those who come to Paris to be cured are more frequently restored than those who inhabit that city. Removed from their former acquaintances, they should be subjected to a regular life and exact discipline, and be treated by all with the utmost kindness and humanity. Their passions should be carefully managed, the fears of the timid should be allayed, and the disconsolate should be consoled. In conversation with them, it is always necessary to speak with truth and sincerity, and never employ other language than that of reason and benevolence.

But no precise rules can be laid down for conducting the moral treatment. Each case of insanity should be studied by itself, and most thoroughly. The history of the individual affected by it should be ascertained, his whole life should be reviewed, every faculty of the mind should be examined and a full knowledge of the whole moral man obtained, and then, a proper course of moral treatment can be suggested, and adopted on some fixed principles.

Conversation, associates and amusements that would be useful to one insane person would be injurious to another, but all require to be treated with constant kindness and respect.

In several of the countries of Europe are many excellent institutions for the comfort and the cure of the insane. In our own there are some not excelled by any in Europe, in fact they appear to be nearly perfect : what they now most require are good personal attendants for the inmates, attendants that are active, vigilant, intelligent and experienced, whose dispositions are amiable and benevolent, and whose manners and feelings are refined and delicate. Such a class of attendants, we hope the conductors of our Institutions for the Insane will endeavor to obtain and to keep, even if the expenses of the Institutions are thereby, at first, considerable increased.

A judicious minister of religion should be attached to each institution, his counsel and instruction will often aid in the cure of some cases. Religious impressions give to the thoughts and affections an energy which is sometimes very useful.

EFFECTS OF MENTAL ATTENTION ON BODILY ORGANS.

Dr. Holland, in his late work already referred to, has a chapter on this subject. But he does little more than mention the fact, that concentrating the attention on a bodily organ, augments the sensations derived from it, and effects more or less its actual state and functions. Considering the great experience of Dr. H. too much of the chapter is occupied with conjectures, queries and metaphysical speculations.

He instances the Dyspeptic and Hypochondriac, whom he says, by fixing their consciousness with morbid intentness on certain organs create in them not merely disordered sensations but often disordered actions. The truth of this every physician will admit.

But it is also true that nearly all local diseases, certainly all the neuroses, may be increased by such attention. I have seen tumours, ulcers, and eruptive diseases increased and perpetuated, solely by mental attention directed to the disordered part.

Diseases of the eyes are thus increased, also diseases of the urinary organs. Bowel affections, particularly diarrhea are aggravated and sometimes caused by mental attention. During the prevalence of the Asiatic Cholera in this country, when every person had heard of the premonitory symptoms, there were but few who did not have some of these symptoms, especially griping pains in the abdomen, flatulence, diarrhea, &c.

In Prisons where the discipline was such as to prevent any communication of intelligence from without, the cholera was not heard of, and did not prevail among the prisoners.

" So strict is the seclusion, says Mr. Crawford,* in the Eastern Penitentiary, Philadelphia, that I found on conversing with the prisoners, that they were not aware of the existence of the cholera which had but a few months before prevailed in Philadelphia.

To their ignorance of the existence of the cholera may doubtless be ascribed in a great measure their preservation from this disease, not a single convict having been attacked by it during the whole period that it prevailed in the city of Philadelphia, although the hospital for the reception of patients was in the neighborhood of the prison. The powerful effect of alarm on the bodily system was singularly illustrated at this period at the Massachusetts State Prison. The chaplain having taken occasion one Sunday, from the pulpit. to advert to the ravages of the cholera, most of the prisoners who composed his congregation were, on retiring to their cells seized

---

* Report of William Crawford, Esq., on the Penitentiaries of the United States, addressed to his Majesty's principal Secretary of State for the home department. 1835, p. 11.

with a complaint which it was greatly feared would lead to, but which happily did not terminate in, malignant cholera."

Some of the disorders of the air passages, of the larynx, trachea and bronchia, are kept up by attention. Some coughs are thus aggravated.

Affections of the fauces and throat are kept up by the same cause. Every one knows that attention to the act of swallowing increases the difficulty of performing it. If there is some soreness of the throat, this attention produces more disordered action, more soreness, and more difficulty in swallowing and speaking. This it has appeared to me, often perpetuates soreness of the fauces and difficulty of speaking, of which clergymen have of late years complained.

Some soreness of the throat and vocal organs is first produced by exposure to cold, not unfrequently by exposure to cold immediately after having exercised these parts by speaking in a warm room. The soreness thus produced will usually subside in a few days by rest, and by the ordinary remedies for a cold and sore throat.

But some few cases, originating from other causes, which I shall hereafter mention, having proved very intractable and difficult of cure, — having caused much suffering and prevented a few individuals from public speaking for a long time, and even in some caused a total loss of voice ; others, when affected with soreness of the throat have become alarmingly apprehensive of a like result. They watch the sensations from the affected parts, perpetually, and examine the throat morning, noon and night, and have others examine it as often, they use various gargles and they diet, and thus a *morbid sensibility* of the parts about the throat is produced, and increased vascular action perpetuated.

Like the pupils who attended Corvisart's **Lectures**
26

on the diseases of the heart, by directing their attention to the pulsations of their own, found, or thought they found them irregular, and themselves laboring under severe disease of this organ.

In some instances I have known the attention of clergymen, when thus affected with soreness of the fauces, and apprehensive of a protracted disease, to be diverted from their complaints by strong mental anxiety, and then recovery rapidly ensued. I have also known severe affection of the throat of the kind alluded to, disregarded by clergymen after a few days of ordinary medication, and have known them to preach with the soreness still upon them, and yet recover rapidly.

As I have said there are some cases of soreness of the throat and loss of voice depending on other causes, that are truly deplorable, often protracted for a long time and not unfrequently incurable. These arise from some affection of the brain, or of the nerves distributed to the organs of the voice. Sometimes the affection of the brain or nerves is only functional, arising from some overwhelming mental emotion, such cases may continue for a considerable time and then suddenly recover. Sometimes they yield suddenly to strong mental emotion, as anger. Laughter cured in one instance.

But in other cases the affection of the brain or nerves, that causes the loss of voice, depends upon some alteration of structure, and may be incurable. The injury of the nerves of voice, which prevents them from duly performing their functions, causes soreness and inflammation of the parts to which they are distributed. Numerous instances of this effect resulting from the injury or division of nerves are given in this work. Happily such cases are rare.

M. Jolly, (*Nouv. Biblioth. medic.*) mentions a case of loss of voice succeding a severe hiccough, and accompanied by circumscribed pain in the back part of the head. He supposed this to result from an affection of the base of the brain or the pneumo-gastric nerves. I have known one case of loss of voice followed by epileptic fits, both affections resulting I presume, from some organic affection of the brain.

But if mental attention causes some bodily affections, may it not cure some? Most certainly. Mr. Hunter, I believe it was, directed a patient who had paralysis of one of the lower limbs and wholly unable to bend the knee, to be placed on a table, with the lower limb hanging over it, and to *will* to move the limb. At first no motion could be produced, but after repeated attempts the will seemed to gain power, and by its exertion alone, the limb could be moved.

The celebrated philosopher Kant, was able to forget, by the strength of *thought*, the pains of gout and other diseases. The mental effort, he says, required great effort of the will and caused the blood to rush to his head, but never failed to afford relief.

The influence of the mind — of mental emotion, in causing and curing disease are altogether too much disregarded by medical men. While grief, fear, remorse,* are as depressing as any measures we ever resort to,

---

* It may be asked if remorse is so injurious to health, why do not prisoners, guilty of great crimes die from this cause? Because they do not feel any remorse. They do not and cannot usually be made to feel guilty — they may say they are so, but a thorough acquaintance with them will convince any one that they scarcely ever feel any remorse. For the correctness of this, I appeal to all those who have long had charge of prisoners, and made careful inquiries on this subject. If a good man could commit a great crime, and be thus imprisoned, I have no doubt remorse would impair his health, if it did not kill him.

hope and faith are more powerful tonics than Bark and Wine. Innumerable are the instances that might be adduced in proof of this. Let the following suffice. When the Plague raged at Messina, in 1743, the second of July, the Tutelar Deity, (Holy Mary, Mother of God,) was taken down and carried in procession through the city. The Plague stopped immediately.

In the life of Lord Chief Justice Holt, says Armstrong, a curious anecdote is recorded. When a young man, Holt had a flow of animal spirits which could not well be restrained, and he happened on one occasion, with some companions, to stop at an inn in the country, where they contracted a debt of such amount that they were unable to defray it. In this dilemma they appealed to Holt to get them out of the scrape. Holt observed that the innkeeper's daughter looked remarkably ill, and was told by her father she had an ague. Hereupon he gathered several plants and mixed them together with a great deal of ceremony. afterwards wrapping them in a piece of parchment, upon which he had scrawled certain letters and marks. The ball thus prepared he hung about the young woman's neck, and the ague did not return. After this, the never-failing doctor offered to discharge the bill, but the gratitude of the landlord refused any such thing, and Holt and his companions departed. When he became Lord Chief Justice a woman was brought before him accused of being a witch. She was the last person tried in England for witchcraft. She made no other defence than that she was in possession of a certain ball which infallibly cured ague. The ball was handed up to the judge, who untied it, and found it to be the same identical ball which he had made in his youthful days for the purpose of curing the woman's ague and paying his own bill.

*The influence of a morbid state of the Brain, in causing
Fever and Inflammation.*

Many of the older medical writers, among whom are
Willis, Chirac, Werlhof, Silvia, and Fracassini, maintain-
ed that inflammation of the brain was the proximate cause
of fever. More recently several modern writers, particularly Clutterbuck, have advanced the same opinion.

I do not believe that inflammation of the brain, (as the
word inflammation is generally used,) is the cause of idiopathic fever. But I do believe, that the brain is the organ primarily affected in this disease. What the exact
nature of this disease of the brain is, we are at present
unable to say. Few die in the early stage of fever, and
in the latter stages other organs than the brain having
become implicated, and numerous remedies administered,
the changes of structure found after death may be, and
probably are, the effects of the disease, or of the remedies,
and do not reveal to us any thing respecting the cause
of the disease or of the organ primarily disordered.

In fever there appears to be at first, a loss or change
of vitality or natural energy of the brain ; — such an
impairment of this organ, such a depression of its powers, that it ceases to supply the other parts of the system
with their due proportion of nervous fluid or energy.
This I think is the first step in fever. This causes the
languor, debility and trembling, the disturbed sleep, impaired intelligence, the stupor and vertigo, the diminished
secretions, shrunken features, &c., observed at the commencement of fevers. After a while reaction takes
place and other symptoms are manifested. But they
mostly result I apprehend from the primary affection of
the brain.

The circulation frequently is aroused into great activi-
26*

ty, and various organs may become inflamed or otherwise affected, not however from original disease of these
organs, but in consequence of the disease of the brain,
which organ has ceased to supply them with nervous
power, essential to the healthy performance of their
functions.

It appears to me surprising that Broussais and
others, should attribute idiopathic fever to disease of
the bowels, either to inflammation of the mucous membrane or to disease of the clustered and solitary glands of
the intestines, or believe that these organs are primarily
affected.

That such appearances are found in the bowels after
death from fever as described by Broussais, Brettonneau,
Louis and others, I have no doubt, I have seen such myself, but I consider them not *causes* but *consequences* of
the disease.

The work of M. Louis is high authority with a large
class of medical men.   The author is certainly entitled to
credit for his industry in collecting and recording facts
and cases, though as it seems to me, to a wearisome and
unnecessary extent.   He also lays claim to the most
careful and rigorous deductions from his facts.   But a
conclusion like the following, appears to me, altogether
incorrect and not warranted by the cases he adduces.

Treating of " *Delirium in patients who died of the typhoid affection,*" he says, " as there was only one lesion
which was constant and always the same in all the subjects, viz., the alteration of the elliptical patches of the
small intestines, we must infer that it is in this last lesion
and not in any other that we must look for the *cause* of
the delirium."*

---

* Anatomical, Pathological and Therapeutic Researches upon the
disease known under the name of Gastro-Enterite, Typhoid Fevers,
&c. By P. J. Louis. vol. ii.

Let it be borne in mind that these examinations of M.
Louis, were of cases in some of which the delirium commenced on the first, fourth and fifth day of the fever,
but which did not terminate in death until sometime after
this.

Now according to the dissections of Brettonneau and
others these lesions of the bowels are not noticeable
in the early period of fever. On the fifth day there is
only a little swelling of the glands of Peyer and Brunner
but no ulceration. Hence it is not probable that these
lesions, found after protracted cases of fever, were the
cause of the delirium that occurred the first day of the
disease. How often delirium occurs in other diseases
and in fevers, where no such lesions are found after
death.

I regard the delirium and the disease of the bowels, as
consequences of a primary affection of the brain. Disease of the brain, probably functional, first exists. This
deranges other organs of the body some more and others less. Delirium ensues, the affection of the other
organs is increased, and then not unfrequently the delirium subsides, but the disease established in the bowels or
elsewhere continues and death ensues.

On examination after death, sometimes but trifling
marks of disease are observed in the brain, while other
parts of the system particularly the bowels are found to
be diseased.

In what is now denominated *Typhoid fever* or *Dothinenteritis*, a sporadic and generally non contagious disease, lesions of the follicles of the small intestines are
said to be usually found. While in *Typhus* fever, or a
fever rarely sporadic and very contagious, these lesions
are never, or very rarely noticed. Dr. Perry of Glas-
gow says they are found in about one in six who die from

typhus, while Dr. Gerhard of Philadelphia and others, think they are always absent in genuine typhus fever.

I have used the words *Typhus* and *Typhoid* as they are used, by most modern writers, to designate different fevers. But I very much doubt whether the diseases to which some writers have given these names are distinct. All the symptoms said to distinguish the one disease from the other I have seen in cases that occurred at the same time, in the same family. It may tend to throw some light upon this subject to give somewhat in detail the history of a fever as it prevailed in two families in this vicinity, during the two last months, October and November 1839, premising however that the same fever has prevailed sporadically this year and for many years past in this region. The instances I have selected are remarkable for the unusual number of cases occurring in one family ; and one of these is very remarkable in this region, for the great fatality that attended it. It is not uncommon however, in fact it is quite common for fever in this city and vicinity, to affect several members of the same family and to prevail much more in certain streets and neighborhoods than in others.

History of a Fever that prevailed in the family of E. Pinney, Esq., of East-Windsor, Conn.

Eight cases originated in this family, and were the first that occurred in that vicinity. The cause of the disease it is not possible at present to determine. Mr. Pinney is a highly respectable and wealthy farmer, his house spacious, beautifully situated, and not surrounded by others.

The ages of the patients were as follows 19, 40, 20, 18, 2, 15, 30, 4. Four were attacked about the first of October, the others a few weeks after. Two died, one aged

30 the other 4. In one that recovered the disease continued above two months, kept up apparently by a tympanitic and irritable state of the bowels with some diarrhea and hemorrhage. The others recovered in from two to four weeks. The deaths occurred in the second week of the fever. In one that died the severity of the disease appeared to be in the bowels, which were very tympanitic, there was also profuse diarrhea. In the other the brain was the organ most affected.

Two of the patients were removed to the adjoining town, the symptoms of their disease I do not know, but two of the attendants on one of them sickened of the same fever.

The others that recovered I saw repeatedly in company with Dr. Gillett the attending physician, Drs. Fuller and Ellsworth of this town also saw the same cases. Their symptoms were quite dissimilar. All of these patents but one, might however, be considered as having Typhoid fever. They had diarrhea and a tympanitic state of the bowels, without marked cerebral symptoms, in fact all the symptoms said to characterize *Typhoid* fever. But the other was a case of genuine *Typhus* fever, this patient had suffusion of the eyes, dusky red aspect of the countenance, extreme stupor and inactivity of the mind without abdominal symptoms. I have never seen a case that exhibited in a more marked form, the symptoms that are said to characterise *Typhus* and to distinguish it from *Typhoid* fever.

The history of the Fever that occurred in the family of Mr. Cornish, is briefly as follows. The family reside in the town of Simsbury ten miles west of East-Windsor, where the fever just described prevailed. In this family every member, seven in number, were attacked with symptoms of fever about the middle of October, and within the same fortnight. The family consisted of

Mr. Cornish, his wife and brother, between the ages of
50 and 60, and four sons between the ages of 22 and 29.
All died. Three of them were removed in the early
part of their illness to different parts of the town. Six
attendants on these patients were attacked with the same
fever and two died. Some of these were attendants
only on those that had been removed. Similar cases of
fever occurred in other parts of the town, in those who
had not visited the Cornish family.

The symptoms were not the same in all. *Ten* had
diarrhœa, *one* profuse hemorrhage from the bowels, me-
teorism in every case but in various degrees. All the
fatal cases had suffusion of the eyes, extreme stupor
and deafness. The deafness in some of the cases lasted
only two or three days.

These symptoms were not manifested in those that
recovered. There was hemorrhage from the nose in all
the cases but three, and these had uterine hemorrhage.
Red spots on the skin were noticed in three cases.

But one was examined after death, and in this the
stomach and bowels only. There were three or four
ulcerated patches in the stomach and extensive softening of its mucous membrane. In the intestines, the elliptical plates and isolated follicles at the lower part of
the small intestines much diseased.

I saw three of the fatal cases a short time previous
to death, they appeared to me cases of *Typhus* fever.
The cases that recovered which I saw, appeared milder,
and corresponded as to symptoms with *Typhoid* fever.

Drs. Shurtleff and Case, of Simsbury, and Dr. Sand-
ford, of Tariffville, were the attending physicians. Several of the cases were also seen by Drs. Fuller and
Sumner of this city.

The extreme fatality of this fever in the first family in
which it occurred produced much excitement and alarm,

Reports were circulated that it had been brought into the town in boxes of rotten cheese, putrid fish, &c. At the request of the authorities of the town, Dr. Fuller and myself visited the town and endeavored to ascertain the cause of the disease. But we learned no facts that threw any light upon it.

From these facts, and others which might be adduced, I am convinced that Typhus and Typhoid fever are the same, varying only in degree, and in the organs affected. In what is called Typhus there is more decided disease of the brain, or of some other organ than the bowels.

In what is called Typhoid, there is more affection of the bowels. Both are seen to prevail at the same time, in the same family, and I presume have the same origin.

Fevers vary as to symptoms in different years. One year the bowels are most affected, in another the brain, the bronchia or some other organs. Some seasons petechiæ are observed in most cases, in other seasons they are scarcely ever witnessed. My own observation corresponds with that of the most experienced physicians in this region with whom I have conversed, in this respect, that fevers of late years have affected the bowels more, and other organs less, than formerly: there has been more abdominal affection, more diarrhœa and a greater tendency to hemorrhage from the bowels. Most of these cases, I have no doubt, are cases of Dothinenteritis, that is, cases of Fever in which there is a morbid state of the mucous follicles of the bowels.

But this fever ought not to be considered as essentially different from that which heretofore prevailed, because the symptoms are in a few respects different and the lesions found on dissection not always the same.

The same lesions of the bowels, viz., redness, swelling, and ulceration of the aggregated follicles of Peyer, and the separate follicles of Brunner, are found after death from diseases that are wholly unlike.

In some cases of fever only redness and swelling of these follicles are found, ulceration not having taken place — but the same redness and swelling have been witnessed after death from scarlatina, and other acute diseases, especially redness and swelling of the follicles of Brunner.*

One of the most constant lesions which was met with in the epidemic cholera, was tumefaction of the intestinal follicles, both the separate and the aggregated.

In phthisis, ulceration of the follicles of the intestines are found similar to those noticed after death from fever. Ulceration of the stomach and bowels have existed for a considerable time without producing any marked symptoms or nothing more than slight symptoms of dyspepsia and occasional diarrhœa.

In some instances of death during convalescence from fever, well marked ulcerations of the bowels have been found, exhibiting no tendency to cicatrization. If the fever depended on the ulcerations, how should convalescence occur, while the ulcerations remained unaltered?

Now when we call to mind that in *Typhus* fever, as understood by late writers, disease of these follicles is rarely though sometimes found, we shall be very reluctant to admit, that our continued fever, by some called Typhoid, by others Typhus, has its primary seat in the follicles of the intestines.

In my subsequent remarks I shall mean by the word *fever*, both *Typhus* and *Typhoid* fever, which I consider the same disease.

That no marks of disease were found in the brain,

---

* Andral, Clinique Medicale, Part iv.

after death from fever in some of the cases adduced by M. Louis is not proof to my mind that disease of this organ did not exist, and even give rise to the disease found in other organs. Functional disorder of the brain certainly existed, and this might be sufficient to produce not only the cerebral symptoms but disorder of other organs. Generally, I apprehend, there is in the early stage of fever, actual disease of the brain, but after other organs, especially the bowels, become considerably affected, the disease of the brain subsides.

But actual disease of the brain is usually found after death from severe fever. Innumerable are the cases that might be adduced in support of this. In the epidemic typhus of the years 1809 and 1812 — 13, I dissected, says Rudolphi, a great number of bodies which had died of that disease, and found hardening of the brain in those who died early, and softening in those that died at a late period. The nerves themselves have been found peculiarly soft and flaccid in those that have died of fever.

That fever is a primary affection of the brain, is supported by the fact that certain mental emotions will produce it. On this subject Dr. Armstrong remarks that, " Fear and Horror are Depressents, and frequently produce congestive fever. I have known a child thrown into an attack of this kind which speedily terminated fatally, by seeing the head of a chicken which had been severed from its body by a knife. The impression which the sight made upon its nervous system was so strong as to produce the attack. You may frequently read in the newspapers of persons dying of fright, and they die of what I call congestive fever.

The collapse which succeeds high mental excitement is frequently followed by the same state.

The sudden communication of any bad news will have

27

a similar effect.   The late Mr. Pott was called in consul-
tation on a surgical case : it was suspected that the patient had stone in the bladder.   Mr. Pott examined him,
found a stone, and abruptly said, I congratulate you on
having your complaint perfectly known, for you may be
cured by an operation.   He observed a remarkable
change in the patient's countenance, and having left him,
went home.   His assistant called in the evening and
found the man dead.

A medical man, then, should be cautious, not only in
his communication, but also in his looks.

I saw in one day two cases of inflammation of the
lungs produced by a thunder-storm."

The same author says, " High Mental Emotions have
a stimulating effect.   The preparations among boys for
set days, with the spirit with which they emulate each
other, frequently produce fever.   I have known fever
arise thus from individuals taking great interest in the
proceedings of public assemblies.   I have known it arise,
too, from anger, a high fit of passion will sometimes produce permanent fever.   In short, any thing which interests the mind so deeply as to excite the heart's action,
may be considered as a stimulant.   I frequently have a
stage of fever from the state of my mind.   If any thing
chance to excite me at about seven o'clock in the evening, my pulse becomes quick, my skin becomes hot, my
face becomes flushed, and then I find I could speak, or
write, or do any thing of which I am capable, better than
at any other period.   This state of excitement goes on
till three or four o'clock in the morning, during which
time I can get no sleep ; and when it goes off, it leaves
me in a state of great exhaustion.   A friend of mine
knows a gentleman who is far advanced in life, who has
a sort of intermittent fever of this kind.   On one day he
is in a state of excitement, on the next in a state of col-

lapse. He is an excellent old man, a good companion, and fond of good company ; and he never invites his friends on the day of collapse, for he knows that then he shall be quite dull; but he invites them on the day of excitement, when he is as merry as possible."

Dr. Hamilton, of Edinburgh, states that in 1821, when there was an epidemic fever in that place, the inmates of the Magdalen Asylum became greatly alarmed by the idea that the fever had been introduced into the Asylum with some clothes that had been sent there to be washed. One girl had been seized with the usual symptoms of fever while at the wash tub. Alarm spread, and within four days twenty-two out of a community of fifty individuals, became stricken with fever. They all appeared. says Dr. H., to be decided cases of idiopathic fever. But Dr. H. did not believe they were, and in decided language, told them that they were yielding to their fears alone. This had a happy effect. Several recovered the same night, and in a few days all were at their usual employments.*

What practitioner who has ever witnessed a dangerous epidemic fever but has seen similar attacks of fever from panic ?

How often we notice fever to attack those who have had much mental suffering. How much more frequently tne fearful, the anxious, and the mentally depressed are attacked by fever when it is epidemic, than those who are not so. The celebrated case cited by Broussais, that of his father, seems to me to have been produced by mental emotion. " The emotion caused by my return," says M. Broussais, " excited occurrences that interrupted our

---

* The Influence of Panic in propagating contagious diseases, by Robert Hamilton, M. D., Edinburgh Trans., Vol. 1.

joy. He could not divest himself of a fatal presenti-
ment that my return would inflict upon him the stroke of
death." He had pain of the head, became totally delirious, but finally recovered, as M. Broussais supposes, by
the application of fifty leeches to the epigastrium.

As I have said, the redness, swelling, and ulceration of
the glands of Peyer and Brunner, so frequently alluded
to by recent writers on fever, in my opinion result from
a primary disease of the brain.

It is a well known fact that the interruption of nervous influence, gives a tendency to inflammation and
ulceration in parts cut off from the brain. Thus con-
cussions and fractures of the spine produce inflammation
of the bladder, and dispose the parts below the seat of
injury to slough from the slightest irritation or pressure.
Mr. Earle cut the ulnar nerve behind the elbow. This
produced not only loss of sensation and of motion, but
disposed the fore arm to constant attacks of inflammation. Five years afterwards these effects still remained
and the temperature of the little finger was four degrees
lower than that of the other.*

After death from injury of the brain, putrefaction of
other parts of the body takes place much more rapidly
than after death from the injury of other organs. So affections of the brain that prevent its supplying every part
with its proper quantity of nervous power disposes the
parts thus cut off to disease.

Ulcers on the brain that have lead to death have been
accompanied by inflammation and ulceration of the mucous membrane of the intestines. Two such cases are
related in the *Archives Generales*, for June, 1825. Not
unfrequently encephalitis is mistaken for Typhoid fever.

---

* Medico Chirurgical Review, Vol. 22nd.

The Dublin Journal, for March, 1836, contains a case of a woman received into the hospital, who had been treated for fever before her reception, and for some time after was considered as laboring under fever. She died, and on dissection extensive cerebral hemorrhage and other disease of the brain was found. " A lady," says Dr. Armstrong, " died of fever who had long complained of pain in the back of her head ; and on examination after death a portion of the cerebellum was found softened, very much like custard-pudding.

A man who was brought into the Fever Hospital had an attack of fever. His respiration was heavy, and his pulse oppressed, and he gradually sunk and died. He had chronic inflammation of the brain for a long time, which was followed by an attack of fever. It was considered to be typhus fever by the medical men who sent him to the Fever Hospital."

After death from insanity ulceration in the intestines is quite frequently observed.

From such facts, and a review of much that has been written upon fever, I am induced to believe that it is primarily an affection of the brain — this affection of the brain disposes other organs of the body to disordered action, which ultimately produces structural disease.

The organs thus secondarily affected, are not always the same, varying with age, habits, climate, seasons of the year, &c., &c.

Treatment — On this subject I have but very little to say. No method is applicable to all cases, neither is there any that is generally beneficial in the fevers of one year, that is certain to be so in the fevers of the next ; but may be decidedly pernicious. In very numerous cases, local blood-letting seems to be beneficial at the commencement of the disease. General bleeding is some-

27*

times but not usually required. Some purgative medicine, is at first, I think, always required ; but continued
purgatives, and emetics, though some seasons they may
be proper and useful, I am convinced from my own
observation, have not been so in the fevers which have
prevailed in this region for the last ten years.

There are not many cases of fever, that do not, especially after the few first days require opiates in some
form. Light nourishment, mild beverages, are necessary at first, and in the after stages of the disease, Wine,
Quinine, and a nourishing diet are required. Symptoms
arise not unfrequently which require blisters and other
remedies not here alluded to.

A vast number of cases require but little or no medicine, or nothing more than a laxative, light nourishment
and repose. Every person affected with fever should be
closely watched, every organ daily examined, and a tendency to local disease guarded against as much as possible. When local disease becomes established, it should
be combatted by common remedies adapted to the age,
habits, &c., of the patient, and to the violence of the
affection.

But nothing is more required in Fever, than attention
to the *morale*. Not only should every thing calculated
to agitate or in any way to disturb the mind of the patient be avoided, but every thing calculated to produce,
thought, or to impose upon him the least mental labor.
I need not enter into details for carrying into effect this,
the most essential part of the treatment of fever. Let
the practitioner, whenever he is called to a patient ill
with fever, ever keep in mind that the brain is diseased
and that its repose is extremely desirable. He will then
carefully guard his patient, and prevent his being injured
by noise, light, company, conversation, &c. He will
quiet all fear, and to the best of his ability inspire hope.

Appendix.

Note A.

SINCE the account of the Sixth Pair of nerves : — the *Abducentes*, was written, the following case of disease, as I suppose of this nerve, has occurred.

Miss S. H. aged four years fell and slightly injured her head. She soon after complained of her head, said it hurt her when she jumped. Soon she became restless, hot and feverish, drowsy and partially deranged. One morning when she awoke the left side was found to be lame, weak, and slightly paralytic. The next day the right eye was observed to turn inwards, and she saw objects double. She soon recovered of the lameness and her general health became good. She was brought to me a few weeks after in consequence of the squinting or turning inwards of the right eye. I considered it to arise from an affection of the sixth nerve of the right side at its origin, which paralysed the right abductor muscle of the eye. The same cause, no doubt, by pressing on the medulla oblongata produced the paralysis of the limbs of the left side of the body.

Cupping the back of the neck, purgatives and low diet affected a cure.

In the August number, for 1839, of the *American Journal of the Medical Siences*, is a very interesting case from a foreign Medical Journal, of Anaesthesia (loss of sensation) in the course of distribution of the Fifth nerve, by Dr. Romberg of Berlin.

A lady received a blow on the occiput which produced a total loss of sensibility of all the parts on the left side, to which the third branch of the fifth pair of nerves was distributed. The sense of taste on the left side of the tongue was entirely obliterated, motion was not disturbed. On dissection the only affection of the nerves found, was confined to the third branch of the fifth pair. At its point of entering the foramen ovale it was surrounded by a reddish vascular tissue and its neurilema was hypertrophied and the nerve itself thickened and diseased.

Note B. page 170.

Dr. Rush states, that the noise of the artillery in a battle of the revolution, destroyed the hearing of one soldier, but restored it in another who had been long deaf.

What are the causes of congenital deafness?

Saunders relates one case illustrative of the cause of congenital deafness. In this the labyrinth was occupied by a soft cheesy substance.

Itard, who has published a voluminous work on the diseases of the ear, mentions two cases of congenital deafness, in which the tympanum was filled with a calcareous deposit; also two others, in which a morbid growth had taken place from the membrane lining that cavity, "Vegetations produites par la membrane qui la tapise;" and a fifth, where a gelatinous secretion occupied not only the tympanum, but also the canals of the labyrinth. He likewise speaks of a child, where the auditory nerve was converted into a substance resembling mucus, and of a man, in whom it was shrivelled up and reduced to a mere thread.

There are also cases of congenital deafness being caused by an extension of the true skin over the membrana tympani, by the presence of polypi in the meatus externus, &c.

Mr. Cox* has within the last two years examined the temporal bones of five children who died in the Asylum for the Deaf and Dumb. In two of these he has detected very palpable deviation from the normal structure.

" The subjects examined were all children who died of strumous diseases of the thoracic and abdominal viscera. In three instances, one or both ears were the seat of scrofulous ulceration, affecting the tympanum and meatus externus with partial destruction of the membrana tympani. In one case, the cavity of the tympanum, together with the mastoid cells, was completely filled with the thick cheesy deposit of scrofula, whilst a similar affection pervaded the whole cancellated structure of the petrous bone. The connexions of the ossicula auditus were destroyed, but the bones themselves remained entire. I merely mention these facts as indicating the strumous habit of body, which I believe prevails very generally among the deaf and dumb; for as these affections could have existed but for a short time previous to death, they can hardly be supposed to have had any connexion with the congenital defect in the organ of hearing."

I may also remark, that in all the cases examined, the petrous portions of the temporal bones exhibited more than the usual varieties of size and shape. In some the

---

* Some Remarks on Malformations of the Internal Ear, being the result of Post Mortem Investigation performed in five cases of Congenital Deafness, by Mr. Edward Cox, Demonstrator of Anatomy at Guy's Hospital.—*Med. Chir. Trans. vol.* xix.

bone was so deficient in particular spots as barely to cover the internal cavities, whilst in others there appeared a preternatural osseous development. In one instance, the petrous bone of a child twelve years old, exceeded in size, hardness, and compactness of structure, that of any adult which I have witnessed.

The malformation which I discovered in two instances, may be described in a few words. It consisted in a partial deficiency of two of the semi-circular canals. The extremities of these tubes opening into the vestibule were perfect, but the central portions were impervious, or rather did not exist at all. In the first case, I had the opportunity of examining the ear from one side only. The vertical and oblique semicircular canals were both impervious at their central portions.

In the second case both ears were examined. On the right side, the middle portions of the oblique and vertical canals were wanting, the bone presenting an appearance like that already described. On the left side, the horizontal and vertical canals exhibited a similar imperfection. The scala tympani likewise was terminated, at its larger extremity, by a bony septum, which separated it from the tympanum, and occupied the situation of the membrane of the fenestra rotunda.

Independently of these malformations and the scrofulous affections of the tympanum, there were no appreciable alterations in any of the five subjects examined. The auditory nerves seemed sound, as did the chorda tympani.

In addition to these two cases of mal-formation I may state a third, which was dissected by my friend Mr. Dalrymple, and is now in his possession. In this instance, the aqueduct of the vestibule was so large as to admit the passage of a small probe, whereas, in the natural state, a fine hair can with difficulty be introduced ino the canal.

In the form of an appendix, Mr. Cock adds another dissection of a child that died at the Asylum.

Not a vestige was to be found of the fenestra rotunda on either side, the usual situation of the membrane being occupied by solid bone. The temporal bones were exceedingly large, although soft and spongy in texture. The cavities were more than usually capacious, and the Eustachian tubes presented a remarkable development, being three or four times larger than common. On one side the aqueduct of the vestibule readily allowed the passage of a large bristle ; on the other side, the canal could not be traced through the bone, although its two extremities were more than usually expanded. Suppuration had taken place in one tympanum."

The very able Report of the Directors of the New-York Institution for the Instruction of the Deaf and Dumb for the year 1836, contains some remarks and statistics on this subject.

It states that, "among the cases of congenital deafness, there have been four in which mal-conformation of the organ of hearing, was the cause. But mal-conformation of this organ, or any of the apparatus connected with it, either external or internal, appears, though quite in opposition to the general opinion, to be by no means a frequent cause of deafness from birth. The case of one individual admitted to the New-York Institution, was a very remarkable one. In the instance alluded to, the *meatus auditorius* or external passage of the ear, was entirely wanting, and the auricle reduced to a small projecting cartilage. The face and head of this individual were otherwise deformed ; nevertheless, there seemed to exist on his part no consequent lack of intellectual capacity. This individual hears imperfectly, on opening his mouth, through the Eustachian tubes; and by this means he has, to a trifling extent, learned to articulate.

In many instances, the deafness of a child has only been discovered after some illness in infancy; and the parents express themselves altogether uncertain whether it had previously existed or not. These we classify as cases of congenital deafness. There is great reason, nevertheless, for the belief, that many cases of deafness, supposed to have existed from birth, have been occasioned by disease; even though the fact may have never been suspected. Still we cannot allow our imaginations to carry us so far, as to make us doubt, whether there is in fact any such thing as congenital deafness at all. Such a doubt has recently been expressed in a respectable quarter. From the fourth circular of the Royal Institution at Paris, just received, we learn that Mr. Du Puget of the Institution of Edgbaston, in England, is convinced " that humidity is the first cause, (of deafness) by deranging the glandular system; that this scrofulous disorder becomes hereditary in families, and, that the humor corrupts the cavities of the ears in infants, so as to produce different degrees of deafness. This is what Mr. Du Puget has observed in the greatest part of the deaf mutes that he has known. The best surgeon of Birmingham, who is a member of the committee of the institution, agrees with Mr. Du Puget; his opinion is, that there exists no deaf mutes from birth, and that this infirmity proceeds from the cause just noted. Mr. Du Puget has communicated this opinion to an able physician and sergeon in Ireland, an ardent friend of the deaf and dumb, who is of the same belief."

Two deaths having occurred in the New-York Institution, dissection took place, with a view to discover how far any alteration might be perceptible to the eye; but notwithstanding the care and attention with which the examination was conducted, nothing unusual could be detected in the appearance of the parts supposed to have been affected."

The following interesting table of the *Causes of accidental deafness, with the number attributed to each*, in from the same Report, and is made up from cases observed at the Institutions for the Deaf and Dumb in Europe and in this country.

1	Scarlet fever,	44
2	Spotted fever,	33
3	Inflammatory fever,	7
4	Nervous fever,	5
5	do. and gathering in ears,	1
6	Brain fever,	4
7	do. do. from dentition,	1
8	do. do. from *coup de soleil*,	1
9	Typhus fever,	3
10	Bilious fever,	1
11	Catarrhal fever,	1
12	Epidemic fever,	1
13	Intermittent fever,	1
14	Arthritic fever,	1
15	Fever not named,	38
16	Fever and fits,	1
17	Convulsions,	24
18	Epileptic fits,	6
19	Colds,	26
20	Measles,	35
21	Gatherings in the head,	15
22	Inflammation in the head,	20
23	Falls,	19
24	Scrofula,	12

28

25 Whooping Cough, ... 12
26 Hydrocephalus, ... 9
27   do.   and whooping cough, . . . 1
28 Measles, mumps and whooping cough,. . . 1
29 Small pox, ... 8
30 Injuries of the head, ... 9
31 Disease (not named) in the head, . . . 4
32   do.   do. in ears. 4
33   do.   do. in throat, . . . 1
34   do.   do. in throat and head, . . 1
35 Disease (not named) of tongue, . . . 1
36 Ulcers, ... 2
37 Falling in the water, ... 3
38 Foreign substances in the ear, . . . 2
39 Itch, ... 2
40 Dentition, ... 2
41 Humors in the head, ... 2
42 Scrofulous opthalmia, ... 1
43 Quinsy, ... 1
44 Peripneumonia, ... 1
45 St. Vitus's dance, ... 1
46 Palsy, ... 1
47 Paralysis, ... 1
48 Syphilis, ... 1
49 Mumps, ... 1
50 Croup, ... 1
51 Inflammation of a limb, ... 1
52 Swelling in neck and gathering in ear, with con-
    vulsions, ... 1
53 Injury of the ear, ... 1
54 Bite of a mad cat, ... 1
55 Swallowing tobacco, ... 1
56   do.   poison laurel, ... 1
57 Disease caused by vermin, ... 1
58 Injurious medical treatment, . . . 1

59	Use of calomel, ...	1
60	Report of a cannon, ...	1
61	Gradual decay of hearing, ...	2
62	Loss of hearing without manifest cause, .	4
63	Diseases and accidents unknown, . . .	398

Total, 787

MENTAL ILLNESS AND SOCIAL POLICY
The American Experience

An Arno Press Collection

Barr, Martin W. Mental Defectives: Their History, Treatment and Training. 1904.

The Beginnings of American Psychiatric Thought and Practice: Five Accounts, 1811-1830. 1973

The Beginnings of Mental Hygiene in America: Three Selected Essays, 1833-1850. 1973

Briggs, L. Vernon, et al. History of the Psychopathic Hospital, Boston, Massachusetts. 1922

Briggs, L. Vernon. Occupation as a Substitute for Restraint in the Treatment of the Mentally Ill. 1923

Brigham, Amariah. An Inquiry Concerning the Diseases and Functions of the Brain, the Spinal Cord, and the Nerves. 1840

Brigham, Amariah. Observations on the Influence of Religion upon the Health and Physical Welfare of Mankind. 1835

Brill, A. A. Fundamental Conceptions of Psychoanalysis. 1921

Bucknill, John Charles. Notes on Asylums for the Insane in America. 1876

Conolly, John. The Treatment of the Insane Without Mechanical Restraints. 1856

Coriat, Isador H. What is Psychoanalysis? 1917

Deutsch, Albert. The Shame of the States. 1948

Dewey, Richard. Recollections of Richard Dewey: Pioneer in American Psychiatry. 1936

Earle, Pliny. Memoirs of Pliny Earle, M. D. with Extracts from his Diary and Letters (1830-1892) and Selections from his Professional Writings (1839-1891). 1898

Galt, John M. The Treatment of Insanity. 1846

Goddard, Henry Herbert. Feeble-mindedness: Its Causes and Consequences. 1926

Hammond, William A. A Treatise on Insanity in Its Medical Relations. 1883

Hazard, Thomas R. Report on the Poor and Insane in Rhode-Island. 1851

Hurd, Henry M., editor. The Institutional Care of the Insane in the United States and Canada. 1916/1917. Four volumes.

Kirkbride, Thomas S. On the Construction, Organization, and General Arrangements of Hospitals for the Insane. 1880

Meyer, Adolf. The Commonsense Psychiatry of Dr. Adolf Meyer: Fifty-two Selected Papers. 1948

Mitchell, S. Weir. Wear and Tear, or Hints for the Overworked. 1887

Morton, Thomas G. The History of the Pennsylvania Hospital, 1751-1895. 1895

Ordronaux, John. Jurisprudence in Medicine in Relation to the Law. 1869

The Origins of the State Mental Hospital in America: Six Documentary Studies, 1837-1856. 1973

Packard, Mrs. E. P. W. Modern Persecution, or Insane Asylums Unveiled, As Demonstrated by the Report of the Investigating Committee of the Legislature of Illinois. 1875. Two volumes in one

Prichard, James C. A Treatise on Insanity and Other Disorders Affecting the Mind. 1837

Prince, Morton. The Unconscious: The Fundamentals of Human Personality Normal and Abnormal. 1921

Putnam, James Jackson. Human Motives. 1915

Russell, William Logie. The New York Hospital: A History of the Psychiatric Service, 1771-1936. 1945

Sidis, Boris. The Psychology of Suggestion: A Research into the Subconscious Nature of Man and Society. 1899

Southard, Elmer E. Shell-Shock and Other Neuropsychiatric Problems Presented in Five Hundred and Eighty-Nine Case Histories from the War Literature, 1914-1918. 1919

Southard, E[lmer] E. and Mary C. Jarrett. The Kingdom of Evils. 1922

Southard, E[lmer] E. and H[arry] C. Solomon. Neurosyphilis: Modern Systematic Diagnosis and Treatment Presented in One Hundred and Thirty-seven Case Histories. 1917

Spitzka, E[dward] C. Insanity: Its Classification, Diagnosis and Treatment. 1887

Supreme Court Holding a Criminal Term, No. 14056. The United States vs. Charles J. Guiteau. 1881/1882. Two volumes

Trezevant, Daniel H. Letters to his Excellency Governor Manning on the Lunatic Asylum. 1854

Tuke, D[aniel] Hack. The Insane in the United States and Canada. 1885

Upham, Thomas C. Outlines of Imperfect and Disordered Mental Action. 1868

White, William A[lanson]. Twentieth Century Psychiatry: Its Contribution to Man's Knowledge of Himself. 1936

Willard, Sylvester D. Report on the Condition of the Insane Poor in the County Poor Houses of New York. 1865